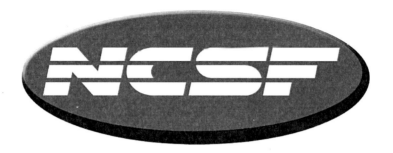

National Council on Strength and Fitness

NCSF Personal Trainer Certification
Workshop Reference Guide

Trademarks:

Document Number 00981216(Rev. A)

© 2012
National Council on Strength & Fitness
PO Box 163908
Miami, FL 33116
Phone 800-772-NCSF • Fax 305-256-7722
Web www.NCSF.org • Email info@ncsf.org

Sports Nutrition Certificate

Table of Contents

Abbreviations in this Manual

Several abbreviations will be used consistently throughout this manual which require your attention. These abbreviations are standard in education and research text.

ADL	Activities of Daily Living
ADP	Adenosine Diphosphate
ATP	Adenosine Triphosphate
(A-V)	Arterio - Venous
BMI	Body Mass Index
BMR	Basal Metabolic Rate
BP	Blood Pressure
BPM	Beats Per Minute
BW	Body Weight
Ca^{++}	Calcium
CAD	Coronary Artery Disease
CHD	Coronary Heart Disease
CHO	Carbohydrate
CO/Q	Cardiac Output
CO_2	Carbon Dioxide
CP	Creatine Phosphate
CRF	Cardiorespiratory Fitness
CV	Cardiovascular
CVD	Cardiovascular Disease
FFM	Fat-Free Mass
DRI	Dietary Reference Intake
HDL	High Density Lipoprotein
HR	Heart Rate
HRR	Heart Rate Reserve
LBP	Low Back Pain
LBW	Lean Body Weight
LDL	Low Density Lipoprotein
O_2	Oxygen
RBP	Resting Blood Pressure
RDA	Recommended Daily Allowance
RHR	Resting Heart Rate
RM	Repetition Maximum
ROM	Range of Motion
RPE	Rate of Perceived Exertion
SV	Stroke Volume
THR	Target/Training Heart Rate
VO_2	Oxygen Consumption
RMR	Resting Metabolic Rate
QOL	Quality of Life

HEALTH SCREENING AND EVALUATION

GENETIC PREDISPOSITION

Uncontrollable factors represent 25-40%, controllable factors – environment/behaviors
- Includes genetic potentials and inherited factors and limitations
- Determines potential capabilities, risks, and physiological occurrence
- Does not preclude health attainment

Learn More: Advanced Concepts of Personal Training Textbook p. 211

METABOLIC SYNDROME

releases ? cytocards

- Central Girth: $\geq$40 inches males, $\geq$35 inches females - *waist*
- Pre-Diabetes: >110 mg/dl fasting blood glucose
- Obesity: $\geq$25% males, $\geq$32% females
- Hypertension: blood pressure >140/90 mmHg
- Hyperlipidemia: high blood lipids (triglycerides and cholesterol)

Learn More: Advanced Concepts of Personal Training Textbook p. 213-222

ETIOLOGY OF COMMON DISEASE

KNOW Guidelines

Cardiovascular Disease (CAD and Stroke)
- Atherosclerosis – build up of plaque in the arterial blood vessels (Stroke, PVD)
- Arteriosclerosis – hardening of the artery reducing vessel elasticity and compliance
- Hypertension – combination of factors leading to excessive peripheral resistance ($\uparrow$BP)
- Hyperlipidemia – elevated blood fats ($\uparrow$ cholesterol/triglycerides)

Diabetes
- Type I – insufficient or no production of insulin – genetic
- Type II – insensitivity to insulin by the cell – behavioral/lifestyle

Learn More: Advanced Concepts of Personal Training Textbook p. 213-222

STRESS CONTINUUM – Total Stress (distress + eustress) vs. Recovery

- Eustress – stress when applied routinely that has a positive adaptive outcome (endorphins)
- Distress – stress associated with negative effects, catabolism, and disease (catecholamines)
- Recovery – the body's process of growth and repair (sleep and nutrients)

Positive	Negative
•Increased neural efficiency	•Increased platelet adhesion
•Increased vascular compliance	•Increased cortisol production
•Increased oxygen extraction	•Increased LDL cholesterol
•Increased cardiac function	•Increased triglycerides
•Increased musculoskeletal tissue integrity and function	•Low-grade inflammation
	•Loss of protein-sparing mechanism

Learn More Advanced Concepts of Personal Training Textbook p. 62

3

INFORMED CONSENT

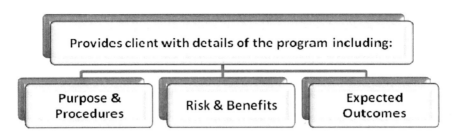

- Most powerful consent in law, but does little to minimize liability when trainer is negligent
- Required documentation for files (includes waiver of liability)

Learn More: Advanced Concepts of Personal Training Textbook p. 235-236

PRACTICE EXERCISE 1: SAMPLE INFORMED CONSENT DOCUMENT

- Read NCSF Workshop Informed Consent - Detect Key Components
- Ask Questions about Physical Participation in the Workshop
- Have a Witness Sign (Meet Your Neighbor)

HEALTH STATUS QUESTIONNAIRE

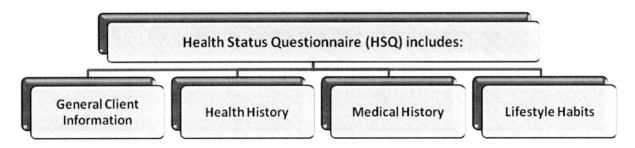

- Useful for self-report data evaluated by a trainer or physician obtained via face-to-face interview (oral administration)
- **Used to make program participation decisions and provide exercise prescription data**
- HSQ: action codes dictate relevance and procedure

Learn More: Advanced Concepts of Personal Training Textbook p. 238

PRACTICE EXERCISES 2 & 3: SAMPLE HEALTH STATUS QUESTIONAIRE & BEHAVIOR FORM
(Case Study part 1)

- **Review HSQ example**
  - ✓ Determine all potential sources of risk obtained via the Self-Report HSQ
  - ✓ Use the action codes to determine participation status and course of action
  - ✓ Participation options: Unrestricted, Supervised, Medically Supervised, Medical Clearance
  - ✓ Document areas to be addressed in the exercise prescription
  - ✓ Correlate the findings on the behavior questionnaire to HSQ findings

HEALTH STATUS QUESTIONNAIRE

SECTION ONE - GENERAL INFORMATION

1. Date: **03/1/2012**

2. Name: **John Delaney**

3. Mailing Address: **15 Elm St. Merribel, PA 18623**   Phone (H): **555-347-2830**

   Phone (W):

   Email: **JMoney@aol.com**

4. *EI* Personal Physician: **Dr. Vincent**   Phone:

   Physician Address: Fax:

5. *EI* Person to contact in case of emergency: **Mary Delaney**   Phone: **Same**

6. Gender (circle one): Female   **Male** *RF*

7. *RF* Date of birth: **06/23/65**

8. Height: **5'10"** Weight: **205 lbs.**

9. Number of hours worked per week: Less than 20   20-40   **41-50**   over 50

10. *SLA* More than 25% of the time at your job is spent (circle all that apply):

    Sitting at desk   Lifting loads   Standing   Walking   Driving
    Risk factor

SECTION TWO - CURRENT MEDICAL INFORMATION

11. Date of last medical physical exam: **06/1/2011**

12. Circle all medicine taken or prescribed within the last 6 months:

Blood thinner *MC*	Epilepsy medication *SEP*	Nitroglycerin *MC*
Diabetic *MC*	Heart rhythm medication *MC*	Other_____
Digitalis *MC*	**High blood pressure medication** *MC*	
Diuretic *MC*	Insulin *MC*	

    need med. clearance

13. Please list any orthopedic conditions. Include any injuries in the last six months.

    ACL tear in High School – Surgically repaired

5

14. Any of these health symptoms that occur frequently (two or more times/month) require medical attention. Please check any that apply.

a. ___ Cough up blood *MC*

g. ___ Swollen joints *MC*

b. ___ Abdominal pain *MC*

h. ___ Feel faint *MC*

c. ___ Low-back pain *MC*

i. ___ Dizziness *MC*

d. ___ Leg pain *MC*

j. ___ Breathlessness with slight exertion *MC*

e. ___ Arm or shoulder pain *MC*

k. ___ Palpitation or fast heart beat *MC*

f. ___ Chest pain *RF MC*

l. ___ Unusual fatigue with normal activity *MC*

Other_____

SECTION THREE - MEDICAL HISTORY

15. Please circle any of the following for which you have been diagnosed or treated by a physician or health professional:

Alcoholism *SEP*	Diabetes *SEP*	Kidney problem *MC*
Anemia, sickle cell *SEP*	Emphysema *SEP*	Mental illness *SEP*
Anemia, other *SEP*	Epilepsy *SEP*	Neck strain *SLA*
Asthma *SEP*	Eye problems *SLA*	Obesity *RF*
Back strain *SLA*	Gout *SLA*	Phlebitis *MC*
Bleeding trait *SEP*	Hearing loss *SLA*	Rheumatoid arthritis *SLA*
Bronchitis, chronic *SEP*	Heart problems *MC*	Stress *RF*
Stroke *MC*	Cancer *SEP*	**High blood pressure** *SLA*
Thyroid problem *SEP*	Cirrhosis *MC*	HIV *SEP*
Ulcer *SEP*	Concussion *MC*	Hypoglycemia *SEP*
Congenital defect *SEP*	Hyperlipidemia *RF*	Other_____

16. Circle any operations that you have had:

Back *SLA*	Heart *MC*	Kidneys *SLA*	Eyes *SLA*	**Joints** *SLA*	Neck *SLA*
Ears *SLA*	Hernia *SLA*	Lungs *SLA*	Other_____		

17. *RF* Circle any of the following who died of heart attack before age 55:

Father   Brother   Son

18. *RF* Circle any of the following who died of heart attack before age 65:

Mother   Sister   Daughter

SECTION FOUR - HEALTH-RELATED BEHAVIORS

19. *RF* Do you currently smoke? Yes   **No**

20. *RF* If you are a smoker, indicate the number smoked per day:

   Cigarettes: 40 or more   20-39   10-19   1-9

   Cigars or pipes only: 5 or more or any inhaled less than 5

21. Have you ever smoked?   Yes   **No**

22. *RF* Do you exercise regularly?   Yes   **No**

23. Last physical fitness test: **High School**

24. How many days a week do you accumulate 30 minutes of moderate activity?

                     0   1   2   3   4   5   6   7

25. How many days per week do you normally spend at least 20 minutes in vigorous exercise?

                     0   1   2   3   4   5   6   7

26. What activities do you engage in a least once per week?   **Golf**

27. Weight now: **205 lbs.**   One year ago: **200 lbs.**   Age 21:   **170 lbs.**

SECTION FIVE - HEALTH-RELATED ATTITUDES

28. These are traits that have been associated with coronary-prone behavior. Circle the number
    that corresponds to how you feel toward the following statement:

                     I am an impatient, time-conscious, hard-driving individual.

                     Circle the number that best describes how you feel:

          6= Strongly agree   3= Slightly disagree
          5= Moderately agree   2= Moderately disagree
          4= Slightly agree   1= Strongly disagree

29. How often do you experience "negative" stress from each of the following?

	RF Always	RF Usually	RF Frequently	Rarely	Never
Work:	_____	_____	X	_____	_____
Home or family:	_____	_____	_____	X	_____
Financial pressure:	_____	_____	_____	X	_____
Social pressure:	_____	_____	_____	X	_____
Personal health:	_____	_____	_____	X	_____

30. List everything not included on this questionnaire that may cause you problems in a fitness test or fitness program.

_____

_____

_____

_____

Action Codes

EI = Emergency Information - must be readily available.

MC = Medical Clearance needed - do not allow exercise without physician's permission.

SEP = Special Emergency Procedures needed - do not let participant exercise alone; make sure the person's exercise partner knows what to do in case of an emergency.

RF = Risk Factor of CHD (educational materials and workshops needed).

SLA = Special or Limited Activities may be needed - you may need to include or exclude specific exercises.

Other (not marked) = Personal information that may be helpful for files or research.

PRACTICE EXERCISES 2 & 3: HEALTH BEHAVIOR FORM REVIEW (Case Study part 2)

Review the following sample client's Behavior Form noting anything that would negatively affect his health. Take into consideration the responses on his HSQ.

BEHAVIOR QUESTIONNAIRE

1. How many servings of fruits and vegetables do you eat per day?

        0   **1**   2   3+

2. How many caffeinated drinks (coffee, tea, cocoa, soft drinks) do you drink per day?

        0   1-2   **3-4**   5+

3. How many glasses (8 ounces) of water do you drink per day?

       0-3   **4-5**   6-7   8+

4. How many meals do you consume per day?

       1-2   **3-4**   5-6   7+

5. I cook with and eat fats:
   - ____ Nearly always cook/eat high fat foods (fried foods, shortening, butter, creams)
   - ____ Cook/eat mostly high fat
   - _X_ Cook/eat both high and low fat foods
   - ____ Cook/eat mostly low fat
   - ____ Cook/eat only low fat

6. My bread/grain eating habit is:
   - ____ Nearly always eat refined (white bread, grains, rolls, crackers, cereal)
   - ____ Eat mostly refined grain products
   - _X_ Eat a mixture of refined and whole grain products
   - ____ Eat primarily whole grain products
   - ____ Eat only whole grain products

7. How often do you eat out?
   - _X_ I eat out nearly every day
   - ____ I eat out several times each week
   - ____ I eat out a few times each month
   - ____ I seldom or never eat out

8. My salty food habit is: (check all that apply)
   - ____ I rarely eat salty foods (chips, pickles, soups, added salt)
   - _X_ Occasionally I eat salty foods
   - ____ I regularly eat salty food
   - ____ I add salt to the foods I eat

9. During the past 30 days, did you diet to lose weight or to keep from gaining weight?

       Yes   **No**

    If Yes Explain: _____

9

10. My high fat snack eating habit is:

          ___ I eat high fat snack foods (potato chips) 3 or more times daily
          ___ I eat high fat snacks once or twice daily
          _X_ I eat high fat snacks a few times each week
          ___ I rarely or never eat high fat snacks

11. How often do you eat red meat?

          ___ I eat red meat nearly every day
          _X_ I eat red meat several times each week
          ___ I eat red meat a few times each month
          ___ I seldom or never eat red meat

12. How often do you eat cookies, cakes, sweets?

          ___ I eat cookies, cakes, sweets nearly every day
          ___ I eat cookies, cakes, sweets several times each week
          _X_ I eat cookies, cakes, sweets a few times each month
          ___ I seldom or never eat cookies, cakes, sweets

13. How many alcoholic beverages do you consume per week?

          0-3   4-5   **6-7**   8+

14. On average, I sleep _____ hours a night.

          3-4   **5-6**   7-8   8+

15. Outside of work, what physical and/or social activities do you engage in?

    Play golf, boating and fishing.

PRACTICE EXERCISES 2 & 3: RESTING MEASURES REVIEW (Case Study part 3)

Resting Heart Rate	80 beats · min^{-1}
Resting Blood Pressure	136/84 mm/Hg
Body Fat	23%
Central Girth	39 inches
BMI	29.4

Category	Medical Referral	Pre-Disease	Healthy Values
Heart rate	100 beats · min^{-1}	90 beats · min^{-1}	<75 beats · min^{-1}
Blood pressure	160/100 mmHg	120/80 -139/89 mmHg	115/75 mmHg
Body Fat	M ≥30% F ≥40%	M 20-24% , F 28-31%	M <19%, F <27%
Total Cholesterol	>240 mg/dl	200-239 mg/dl	<200 mg/dl

any of these need a medical referral

ASSESSING COMPONENTS OF FITNESS

Health Related Components

Cardiovascular Fitness - The body's ability to efficiently use oxygen; quantified by maximal aerobic capacity (VO_2max). Correlates with general lifespan and is inversely associated with risk of CVD. Assessed using submax and max tests - GXT, run/walk tests, step tests, cycle ergometer, etc.

Muscular Strength - Primary component of Muscular Fitness. Defined by a **maximal contractile force of a muscle or muscle group.** Muscle specific - affected by the movement system including stabilizers and neutralizers. Associated with general function, musculoskeletal disease risk, risk of injuries, and living quality. Assessed using 1RM, 3RM, and multi-rep tests.

Muscular Endurance - Secondary component of Muscular Fitness and associated with muscular strength (i.e., a 200 lb power lifter will be able to carry a heavy piece of furniture further than a 150 lb marathon runner). Assessed by the **rate of decline of a muscle's force production** - repeated contractile force output of prime movers and stabilizers. Correlates with living quality and musculoskeletal health. Assessed using prolonged rep or time to failure tests such as abdominal curl-up or arm hang.

Body Composition - A person's relative leanness, ratio of body fat to fat-free mass (expressed as a percentage). Strongly associated with risk of metabolic disease and CVD. Metabolic fitness is often included with this category - addresses quantity of lean mass and behaviors affecting metabolism. Assessed using skinfold, girth measures, hydrostatic weighing, and bioelectric impedance.

Flexibility - **Joint specific range of motion.** Correlates with movement function, bodily pain, and musculoskeletal and joint health. Key factor is viscoelasticity of muscle connective tissue (fascia). Reductions with age-associated decreased activity and reduced hydration of tissue. Assessed by movement screens and goniometer measurements.

Performance Related Components

Power - Muscle Power = **Muscle Force x Muscle Contractile Velocity** With age there is a selective atrophy of Type II (powerful) motor units which reduces functional activities (e.g. getting up from a chair requires a powerful and quick hip extending contraction). Assessed using vertical jump, MB throws, speed tests, or chair stands.

Agility - **Ability to efficiently change direction; accelerate and decelerate movements,** quick moving, quick stopping. Critical in sports performance movement efficiency. Important for functional performance in negotiating obstacles and maintaining mobility in multiple-planes. Assessed using 20 yd shuttle or timed cone courses.

Coordination - **Ability to efficiently perform a task integrating movements of the body.** Synchronicity of neuromuscular recruitment patterns. Motor unit coordination contributes to force production during a skill or task. Assessed using performance criteria during certain movements.

Speed - **The time it takes to move a given distance.** Movement speed is inversely related to force, but an important component of power. Correlates with sports performance and functionality. Gait speed is a reliable predictor of fall risk in the elderly (faster gait = less risk of falling) and correlates with mobility. Assessed using running distances.

Balance - **Ability to maintain static stability (equilibrium) or move without falling.** Correlates strongly with sports performance, geriatric fall risk and movement speed. Improves stability, enabling greater force production. Assessed using Bapse boards or other balance devices.

Learn More: Advanced Concepts of Personal Training Textbook p. 207-211

CREATE A NEEDS ANALYSIS

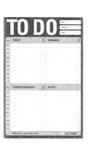

- Assess and list signs/symptoms of disease and health limitations based on screening
- Determine additional need based on resting and active physical testing battery
- List limitations associated with health/fitness deficiencies
- Identify behavior factors that contribute to health issues or present as obstacles to health
- Place the needs in the appropriate training category by order of importance

Learn More: Advanced Concepts of Personal Training Textbook p. 255-256

GOAL ATTAINMENT

- Planned structure of quantifiable steps to change behavior
- **Objectives** – daily actions needed to meet short-term goal – quantify/assign
- **Short-term goal** – generally less than one month – collective objectives
- **Long-term goal** – sustained completion of short-term goals

Learn More: Advanced Concepts of Personal Training Textbook p. 256-257

PROGRAM DEVELOPMENT

- Use program activities that address the needs list
- Program activities should attempt to **address multiple areas of need simultaneously**
- Premeditate program activities with specific outcome goals with intended completion dates

Learn More: Advanced Concepts of Personal Training Textbook p. 485

BODY COMPOSITION AND WEIGHT MANAGEMENT

BODY COMPOSITION

Body composition is the ratio of Fat Mass (FM) to Fat-Free Mass (FFM)

- **Visceral Fat**: Fat stored between, in, and around organs *most dangerous for disease*
- **Subcutaneous Fat**: Fat stored between the skin and muscle
- **Intramuscular Fat**: Fat stored within muscle tissue
- **Fat-Free Mass**: Muscles, bones, connective tissue, and water

FFM is more dense than FM. Hydration status is a major component of FFM; muscle mass is ≈70% water, fat mass ≈50%.

Some fat mass **(essential body fat)** is needed for protection of organs, insulation, energy stores, hormonal balance, and as a component of nerve and cell membranes.

Essential Body Fat - represents lowest limits of body fat necessary for maintaining good health.

hazardous

3-5% body fat for males (key issue: temperature regulation)
11-14% body fat females (key issue: hormonal, amenorrhea)

	Essential	Lean/Fit	Healthy	Risk	Obesity
Males	**3-5%**	6-15%	16-19%	20-24%	≥25%
Females	**11-14%**	15-22%	23-26%	27-31%	≥32%

hazardous

Learn More: Advanced Concepts of Personal Training Textbook p. 169-171

FAT CELL STORAGE

Regional Fat Distribution - amount and site vary based upon genetic predisposition and gender.

Gynoid storage – (Women) fat stored predominately in the thighs, buttocks, and hips. It is characterized by hypertrophy/hyperplasia of fat cells and has limited metabolic activity due to low hormone-receptor density.

Android storage – (Men) predominantly have androgenic-associated (male hormone) fat storage that predominates in the abdomen and back. It is characterized by hyperinsulinemia, increased levels of LDL-cholesterol, high triglycerides, and hypertension. The fat is metabolically active due to a higher concentration of adrenal-sensitive, beta receptors.

• Central adiposity; highly metabolic;

Waist-to-Hip Ratio (WHR) estimates the extent of android obesity. Abdominal circumference alone (≥35 inches for female and ≥40 inches for male) can be used to estimate disease risk.

Body Mass Index (BMI) provides a value reflecting propensity for disease based on weight ÷ height^2.

Learn More: Advanced Concepts of Personal Training Textbook p. 170 & 175

13

EVALUATION OF BODY FAT

BODY COMPOSITION: METHODS OF ASSESSMENT

Method	Advantage/Limitation	Description
Girth Measurement	Easy methodology Reduced accuracy for muscular individuals SEE 4% with regression equation	Circumference measures are used to calculate body composition. Can be used effectively with obese individuals.
Hydrostatic Weighing	Accurate, expensive, not practical in most settings	Based on Archimedes principle. Displacement is used in calculating the body mass density & percent fat.
Bioelectrical Impedance	Easy methodology Accuracy limited by instrument and testing parameters	Lean tissue is electrically conductive, fat mass is not. Limited by water balance, electrolyte levels, skin temperature and thickness.
Skinfold Measurement	Accurate - SEE up to 4% Limited by tester accuracy	Measures the thickness of skinfolds based on the fact that 50%-70% of fat lies directly under skin. Skinfold sites vary and are specific to the formula used to calculate percentage of fat.

* SEE = Standard Estimation of Error

Learn More: Advanced Concepts of Personal Training Textbook p. 176-184

PRACTICE EXERCISE 4: GIRTH MEASUREMENTS

Using a partner as a sample client, perform the following girth estimation of body fat percentage. Be able to describe some potential sources of weakness for this method and for what populations this would be best served. Textbook pages 293-294 show the anatomical locations where measurements should be taken.

2-3 GIRTH BODY FAT ESTIMATION

The 2-3 girth method of body fat estimation can also be a viable option to predict body fat, particularly when working with the obese population and accurate caliper readings cannot be made. The advantage of the 2-3 girth measurement is the assessment utilizes two circumference values for men and 3 circumference values for women to estimate body fat. This may reduce the *SEE* compared to other assessments when determining body composition. The standard estimation of error is about 3.5%.

Calculating your 2-3 girth measurement requires the use of Tables A and B on the following pages. The percent body fat can be found by using the derived circumference value (inches) and identifying the percent fat score that corresponds to the calculated value from the circumference measurements.

Step #1   Measure the appropriate anatomical positions.

Men   Abdominal girth circumference *belly button*   _____32_____ in.

Neck circumference   _____14 ~~18~~_____ in.

below adams apple

Women   Upper abdominal circumference *2 in above belly button*   _____ in.

Hip circumference   _____ in.

Neck circumference   _____ in.

Step #2   Find the derived circumference value (CV)

Men: (__32__ Abdominal – __14__ Neck) = __18__ CV   *5'9" = 16%*

Women: (_____ Upper abdominal + _____ Hip) = _____ – _____ Neck = _____ CV

Enter your derived Circumference Value (CV) here   _____

Step #3   Use the following tables (**Table A for Men** and **Table B for Women**) to find the estimated body fat % by matching the derived circumference value in the left hand column with your height in inches across the top.

Enter your 2-3 Girth body fat estimation here   _____%

Circumference value (in)	TABLE A Men's BF % 2-3 Girth									
	HEIGHT (IN)									
	60.0	60.5	61	61.5	62	62.5	63	63.5	64	64.5
11	3	2	2	2	2	1	1	1	1	1
11.5	4	4	4	3	3	3	3	2	2	2
12	6	5	5	5	5	4	4	4	4	3
12.5	7	7	6	6	6	6	6	5	5	5
13	8	8	8	8	7	7	7	7	6	6
13.5	10	9	9	9	9	8	8	8	8	8
14	11	11	10	10	10	10	10	9	9	9
14.5	12	12	12	11	11	11	11	11	10	10
15	13	13	13	13	12	12	12	12	12	11
15.5	15	14	14	14	14	13	13	13	13	12
16	16	15	15	15	15	15	14	14	14	14
16.5	17	17	16	16	16	16	15	15	15	15
17	18	18	17	17	17	17	16	16	16	16
17.5	19	19	19	18	18	18	18	17	17	17
18	20	20	20	19	19	19	19	18	18	18
18.5	21	21	21	20	20	20	20	19	19	19
19	22	22	22	21	21	21	21	20	20	20
19.5	23	23	23	22	22	22	22	21	21	21
20	24	24	23	23	23	23	22	22	22	22
20.5	25	25	24	24	24	24	23	23	23	23
21	26	26	25	25	25	25	24	24	24	24
21.5	27	26	26	26	26	25	25	25	25	24
22	28	27	27	27	27	26	26	26	26	25
22.5	28	28	28	28	27	27	27	27	26	26
23	29	29	29	29	28	28	28	28	27	27
23.5	30	30	30	29	29	29	29	28	28	28
24	31	31	30	30	30	30	29	29	29	29
24.5	32	31	31	31	31	30	30	30	30	29
25	33	32	32	32	31	31	31	31	30	30
25.5	33	33	33	33	32	32	32	31	31	31
26	34	34	34	33	33	33	32	32	32	32
26.5	35	35	34	34	34	33	33	33	33	32
27	36	35	35	35	34	34	34	34	33	33
27.5	36	36	36	35	35	35	35	34	34	34
28	37	37	36	36	36	36	35	35	35	35
28.5	38	37	37	37	37	36	36	36	36	35
29	38	38	38	38	37	37	37	37	36	36
29.5	39	39	39	38	38	38	37	37	37	37
30	40	39	39	39	39	38	38	38	38	37
30.5	-	-	40	40	39	39	39	39	38	38
31	-	-	-	-	40	40	39	39	39	39
31.5	-	-	-	-	-	-	-	40	40	39
32.0-35.0	-	-	-	-	-	-	-	-	-	40

TABLE A Men's BF % 2-3 Girth									
HEIGHT (IN)									
Circumference value (in)	65	65.5	66	66.5	67	67.5	68	68.5	69	69.5
11	0	0	-	-	-	-	-	-	-	-
11.5	2	2	1	1	1	1	1	0	0	-
12	3	3	3	3	2	2	2	2	2	1
12.5	5	4	4	4	4	4	3	3	3	3
13	6	6	6	5	5	5	5	5	4	4
13.5	7	7	7	7	6	6	6	6	6	5
14	9	8	8	8	8	8	7	7	7	7
14.5	10	10	9	9	9	9	9	8	8	8
15	11	11	11	10	10	10	10	10	9	9
15.5	12	12	12	12	11	11	11	11	11	10
16	13	13	13	13	12	12	12	12	12	11
16.5	14	14	14	14	14	13	13	13	13	13
17	16	15	15	15	15	14	14	14	14	14
17.5	17	16	16	16	16	16	15	15	15	15
18	18	17	17	17	17	17	16	16	16	16
18.5	19	18	18	18	18	18	17	17	17	17
19	20	19	19	19	19	19	18	18	18	18
19.5	21	20	20	20	20	19	19	19	19	19
20	22	21	21	21	21	20	20	20	20	20
20.5	22	22	22	22	22	21	21	21	21	20
21	23	23	23	23	22	22	22	22	22	21
21.5	24	24	24	24	23	23	23	23	22	22
22	25	25	25	24	24	24	24	24	23	23
22.5	26	26	25	25	25	25	25	24	24	24
23	27	27	26	26	26	26	25	25	25	25
23.5	28	27	27	27	27	26	26	26	26	26
24	28	28	28	28	27	27	27	27	27	26
24.5	29	29	29	29	28	28	28	28	27	27
25	30	30	30	29	29	29	29	28	28	28
25.5	31	31	30	30	30	30	29	29	29	29
26	32	31	31	31	31	30	30	30	30	29
26.5	32	32	32	32	31	31	31	31	30	30
27	33	33	32	32	32	32	32	31	31	31
27.5	34	33	33	33	33	33	32	32	32	32
28	34	34	34	34	33	33	33	33	33	32
28.5	35	35	35	34	34	34	34	33	33	33
29	36	36	35	35	35	35	34	34	34	34
29.5	36	36	36	36	35	35	35	35	35	34
30	37	37	37	36	36	36	36	35	35	35
30.5	38	38	37	37	37	37	36	36	36	36
31	38	38	38	38	37	37	37	37	37	36
31.5	39	39	39	38	38	38	38	37	37	37
32	40	39	39	39	39	38	38	38	38	38
32.5	-	-	40	40	39	39	39	39	38	38
33	-	-	-	-	40	40	39	39	39	39
33.5	-	-	-	-	-	-	-	40	40	39
34	-	-	-	-	-	-	-	-	-	40
34.5	-	-	-	-	-	-	-	-	-	-
35.0	-	-	-	-	-	-	-	-	-	-

	TABLE A Men's BF % 2-3 Girth									
	HEIGHT (IN)									
Circumference value (in)	70	70.5	71	71.5	72	72.5	73	73.5	74	74.5
11	-	-	-	-	-	-	-	-	-	-
11.5	-	-	-	-	-	-	-	-	-	-
12	1	1	1	1	0	0	0	-	-	-
12.5	3	2	2	2	2	2	1	1	1	1
13	4	4	4	3	3	3	3	3	2	2
13.5	5	5	5	5	4	4	4	4	4	4
14	7	6	6	6	6	6	5	5	5	5
14.5	8	8	7	7	7	7	7	6	6	6
15	9	9	9	8	8	8	8	8	7	7
15.5	10	10	10	9	9	9	9	9	9	8
16	11	11	11	11	10	10	10	10	10	9
16.5	12	12	12	12	12	11	11	11	11	11
17	13	13	13	13	13	12	12	12	12	12
17.5	14	14	14	14	14	13	13	13	13	13
18	15	15	15	15	15	14	14	14	14	14
18.5	16	16	16	16	16	15	15	15	15	15
19	17	17	17	17	17	16	16	16	16	16
19.5	18	18	18	18	18	17	17	17	17	17
20	19	19	19	19	18	18	18	18	18	17
20.5	20	20	20	20	19	19	19	19	19	18
21	21	21	21	20	20	20	20	20	19	19
21.5	22	22	22	21	21	21	21	21	20	20
22	23	23	22	22	22	22	22	21	21	21
22.5	24	23	23	23	23	23	22	22	22	22
23	25	24	24	24	24	23	23	23	23	23
23.5	25	25	25	25	24	24	24	24	24	23
24	26	26	26	25	25	25	25	25	24	24
24.5	27	27	26	26	26	26	26	25	25	25
25	28	27	27	27	27	27	26	26	26	26
25.5	28	28	28	28	28	27	27	27	27	27
26	29	29	29	29	28	28	28	28	27	27
26.5	30	30	29	29	29	29	29	28	28	28
27	31	30	30	30	30	30	29	29	29	29
27.5	31	31	31	31	30	30	30	30	30	29
28	32	32	32	31	31	31	31	31	30	30
28.5	33	33	32	32	32	32	31	31	31	31
29	33	33	33	33	33	32	32	32	32	31
29.5	34	34	34	33	33	33	33	33	32	32
30	35	35	34	34	34	34	33	33	33	33
30.5	35	35	35	35	35	34	34	34	34	33
31	36	36	36	35	35	35	35	34	34	34
31.5	37	36	36	36	36	36	35	35	35	35
32	37	37	37	37	36	36	36	36	36	35
32.5	38	38	37	37	37	37	37	36	36	36
33	39	38	38	38	38	37	37	37	37	37
33.5	39	39	39	38	38	38	38	38	37	37
34	40	39	39	39	39	39	38	38	38	38
34.5	-	-	40	40	39	39	39	39	39	38
35.0	-	-	-	-	40	40	40	39	39	39

TABLE A Men's BF % 2-3 Girth										
	HEIGHT (IN)									
Circumference value (in)	75	75.5	76	76.5	77	77.5	78	78.5	79	79.5
11	-	-	-	-	-	-	-	-	-	-
11.5	-	-	-	-	-	-	-	-	-	-
12	-	-	-	-	-	-	-	-	-	-
12.5	1	1	0	0	-	-	-	-	-	-
13	2	2	2	1	1	1	1	1	1	0
13.5	3	3	3	3	3	2	2	2	2	2
14	5	4	4	4	4	4	3	3	3	3
14.5	6	6	5	5	5	5	5	5	4	4
15	7	7	7	6	6	6	6	6	6	5
15.5	8	8	8	8	7	7	7	7	7	6
16	9	9	9	9	8	8	8	8	8	8
16.5	10	10	10	10	10	9	9	9	9	9
17	11	11	11	11	11	10	10	10	10	10
17.5	12	12	12	12	12	11	11	11	11	11
18	13	13	13	13	13	12	12	12	12	12
18.5	14	14	14	14	14	13	13	13	13	13
19	15	15	15	15	15	14	14	14	14	14
19.5	16	16	16	16	16	15	15	15	15	15
20	17	17	17	17	16	16	16	16	16	16
20.5	18	18	18	18	17	17	17	17	17	16
21	19	19	19	18	18	18	18	18	18	17
21.5	20	20	20	19	19	19	19	19	18	18
22	21	21	20	20	20	20	20	19	19	19
22.5	22	21	21	21	21	21	20	20	20	20
23	22	22	22	22	22	21	21	21	21	21
23.5	23	23	23	23	22	22	22	22	22	21
24	24	24	24	23	23	23	23	23	22	22
24.5	25	25	24	24	24	24	24	23	23	23
25	26	25	25	25	25	25	24	24	24	24
25.5	26	26	26	26	26	25	25	25	25	25
26	27	27	27	26	26	26	26	26	25	25
26.5	28	28	27	27	27	27	27	26	26	26
27	28	28	28	28	28	27	27	27	27	27
27.5	29	29	29	29	28	28	28	28	28	27
28	30	30	29	29	29	29	29	28	28	28
28.5	31	30	30	30	30	30	29	29	29	29
29	31	31	31	31	30	30	30	30	30	29
29.5	32	32	31	31	31	31	31	30	30	30
30	33	32	32	32	32	32	31	31	31	31
30.5	33	33	33	33	32	32	32	32	32	31
31	34	34	33	33	33	33	33	32	32	32
31.5	34	34	34	34	34	33	33	33	33	33
32	35	35	35	34	34	34	34	34	33	33
32.5	36	35	35	35	35	35	34	34	34	34
33	36	36	36	36	35	35	35	35	35	34
33.5	37	37	36	36	36	36	36	35	35	35
34	37	37	37	37	37	36	36	36	36	36
34.5	38	38	38	37	37	37	37	37	36	36
35.0	39	38	38	38	38	38	37	37	37	37
35.5	39	39	39	39	38	38	38	38	38	37
36	40	40	39	39	39	39	39	38	38	38
36.5	-	-	40	40	39	39	39	39	39	38
37	-	-	-	-	-	40	40	39	39	39
37.5	-	-	-	-	-	-	-	40	40	40
38	-	-	-	-	-	-	-	-	-	-
38.5	-	-	-	-	-	-	-	-	-	-

Circumference value (in)	58	58.5	59	59.5	60	60.5	61	61.5	62	62.5
TABLE B Women's BF % 2-3 Girth										
HEIGHT (IN)										
34.5	1	0	-	-	-	-	-	-	-	-
35	2	1	1	1	0	-	-	-	-	-
35.5	3	2	2	2	1	1	0	0	-	-
36	4	3	3	3	2	2	1	1	1	0
36.5	5	4	4	4	3	3	2	2	2	1
37	6	5	5	4	4	4	3	3	3	2
37.5	7	6	6	5	5	5	4	4	4	3
38	7	7	7	6	6	6	5	5	5	4
38.5	8	8	8	7	7	7	6	6	5	5
39	9	9	9	8	8	7	7	7	6	6
39.5	10	10	9	9	9	8	8	8	7	7
40	11	11	10	10	10	9	9	8	8	8
40.5	12	12	11	11	10	10	10	9	9	9
41	13	12	12	12	11	11	11	10	10	10
41.5	14	13	13	13	12	12	11	11	11	10
42	14	14	14	13	13	13	12	12	12	11
42.5	15	15	15	14	14	13	13	13	12	12
43	16	16	15	15	15	14	14	14	13	13
43.5	17	17	16	16	15	15	15	14	14	14
44	18	17	17	17	16	16	16	15	15	14
44.5	19	18	18	17	17	17	16	16	16	15
45	19	19	19	18	18	17	17	17	16	16
45.5	20	20	19	19	19	18	18	18	17	17
46	21	20	20	20	19	19	19	18	18	18
46.5	22	21	21	20	20	20	19	19	19	18
47	22	22	22	21	21	20	20	20	19	19
47.5	23	23	22	22	22	21	21	21	20	20
48	24	23	23	23	22	22	22	21	21	21
48.5	25	24	24	23	23	23	22	22	22	21
49	25	25	25	24	24	23	23	23	22	22
49.5	26	26	25	25	24	24	24	23	23	23
50	27	26	26	26	25	25	24	24	24	23
50.5	27	27	27	26	26	26	25	25	24	24
51	28	28	27	27	27	26	26	25	25	25
51.5	29	28	28	28	27	27	27	26	26	25
52	29	29	29	28	28	28	27	27	27	26
52.5	30	30	29	29	29	28	28	28	27	27
53	31	30	30	30	29	29	29	28	28	27
53.5	31	31	31	30	30	30	29	29	28	28
54	32	32	31	31	31	30	30	30	29	29
54.5	33	32	32	32	31	31	31	30	30	29
55	33	33	33	32	32	32	31	31	30	30
55.5	34	34	33	33	33	32	32	31	31	31
56	35	34	34	33	33	33	32	32	32	31
56.5	35	35	34	34	34	33	33	33	32	32
57	36	35	35	35	34	34	34	33	33	33
57.5	36	36	36	35	35	35	34	34	34	33
58	37	37	36	36	36	35	35	35	34	34
58.5	38	37	37	37	36	36	35	35	35	34
59	38	38	38	37	37	36	36	36	35	35
59.5	39	38	38	38	37	37	37	36	36	36
60	39	39	39	38	38	38	37	37	37	36
60.5	40	40	39	39	39	38	38	37	37	37
61	41	40	40	39	39	39	38	38	38	37
61.5	41	41	40	40	40	39	39	39	38	38
62	42	41	41	41	40	40	40	39	39	38
62.5	42	42	42	41	41	40	40	40	39	39
63	43	42	42	42	41	41	41	40	40	40

TABLE B Women's BF % 2-3 Girth

Circumference value (in)	HEIGHT (IN)									
	63	63.5	64	64.5	65	65.5	66	66.5	67	67.5
34.5	-	-	-	-	-	-	-	-	-	-
35	-	-	-	-	-	-	-	-	-	-
35.5	-	-	-	-	-	-	-	-	-	-
36	0	-	-	-	-	-	-	-	-	-
36.5	1	1	0	-	-	-	-	-	-	-
37	2	2	1	1	1	0	-	-	-	-
37.5	3	3	2	2	2	1	1	1	0	-
38	4	3	3	3	2	2	2	1	1	1
38.5	5	4	4	4	3	3	3	2	2	2
39	6	5	5	5	4	4	4	3	3	3
39.5	7	6	6	6	5	5	5	4	4	4
40	7	7	7	6	6	6	5	5	5	4
40.5	8	8	8	7	7	7	6	6	6	5
41	9	9	8	8	8	7	7	7	6	6
41.5	10	10	9	9	9	8	8	8	7	7
42	11	10	10	10	9	9	9	8	8	8
42.5	12	11	11	11	10	10	10	9	9	9
43	12	12	12	11	11	11	10	10	10	9
43.5	13	13	13	12	12	12	11	11	11	10
44	14	14	13	13	13	12	12	12	11	11
44.5	15	15	14	14	14	13	13	13	12	12
45	16	15	15	15	14	14	14	13	13	13
45.5	16	16	16	15	15	15	14	14	14	13
46	17	17	17	16	16	16	15	15	15	14
46.5	18	18	17	17	17	16	16	16	15	15
47	19	18	18	18	17	17	17	16	16	16
47.5	19	19	19	18	18	18	17	17	17	16
48	20	20	20	19	19	18	18	18	18	17
48.5	21	21	20	20	20	19	19	19	18	18
49	22	21	21	21	20	20	20	19	19	19
49.5	22	22	22	21	21	21	20	20	20	19
50	23	23	22	22	22	21	21	21	20	20
50.5	24	23	23	23	22	22	22	21	21	21
51	24	24	24	23	23	23	22	22	22	21
51.5	25	25	24	24	24	23	23	23	22	22
52	26	25	25	25	24	24	24	23	23	23
52.5	26	26	26	25	25	25	24	24	24	23
53	27	27	26	26	26	25	25	25	24	24
53.5	28	27	27	27	26	26	26	25	25	25
54	28	28	28	27	27	27	26	26	26	25
54.5	29	29	28	28	28	27	27	27	26	26
55	30	29	29	29	28	28	28	27	27	27
55.5	30	30	30	29	29	29	28	28	28	27
56	31	31	30	30	30	29	29	29	28	28
56.5	32	31	31	31	30	30	30	29	29	29
57	32	32	32	31	31	31	30	30	30	29
57.5	33	32	32	32	31	31	31	30	30	30
58	33	33	33	32	32	32	31	31	31	30
58.5	34	34	33	33	33	32	32	32	31	31
59	35	34	34	34	33	33	33	32	32	32
59.5	35	35	35	34	34	34	33	33	33	32
60	36	35	35	35	34	34	34	33	33	33
60.5	36	36	36	35	35	35	34	34	34	33
61	37	37	36	36	36	35	35	35	34	34
61.5	38	37	37	37	36	36	36	35	35	35
62	38	38	37	37	37	36	36	36	35	35
62.5	39	38	38	38	37	37	37	36	36	36
63	39	39	39	38	38	38	37	37	37	36

TABLE B Women's BF % 2-3 Girth

Circumference value (in)	HEIGHT (IN)									
	63	63.5	64	64.5	65	65.5	66	66.5	67	67.5
64	40	40	40	39	39	39	38	38	38	37
64.5	41	41	40	40	40	39	39	39	38	38
65	41	41	41	40	40	40	39	39	39	38
65.5	42	42	41	41	41	40	40	40	39	39
66	43	42	42	41	41	41	40	40	40	39
66.5	43	43	42	42	42	41	41	41	40	40
67	44	43	43	43	42	42	41	41	41	41
67.5	44	44	43	43	43	42	42	42	41	41
68	45	44	44	44	43	43	43	42	42	42
68.5	-	45	44	44	44	43	43	43	42	42
69	-	-	45	45	44	44	44	43	43	43
69.5	-	-	-	-	45	44	44	44	43	43
70	-	-	-	-	-	45	45	44	44	44
70.5	-	-	-	-	-	-	-	45	44	44
71.0-75.5	-	-	-	-	-	-		-	45	45

TABLE B Women's BF % 2-3 Girth

Circumference value (in)	HEIGHT (IN)									
	68	68.5	69	69.5	70	70.5	71	71.5	72	72.5
34.5	-	-	-	-	-	-	-	-	-	-
35	-	-	-	-	-	-	-	-	-	-
35.5	-	-	-	-	-	-	-	-	-	-
36	-	-	-	-	-	-	-	-	-	-
36.5	-	-	-	-	-	-	-	-	-	-
37	-	-	-	-	-	-	-	-	-	-
37.5	-	-	-	-	-	-	-	-	-	-
38	0	0	-	-	-	-	-	-	-	-
38.5	1	1	1	0	0	-	-	-	-	-
39	2	2	2	1	1	1	0	0	-	-
39.5	3	3	3	2	2	2	1	1	1	0
40	4	4	3	3	3	3	2	2	2	1
40.5	5	5	4	4	4	3	3	3	2	2
41	6	5	5	5	5	4	4	4	3	3
41.5	7	6	6	6	5	5	5	4	4	4
42	8	7	7	7	6	6	6	5	5	5
42.5	8	8	8	7	7	7	6	6	6	6
43	9	9	9	8	8	8	7	7	7	6
43.5	10	10	10	9	9	8	8	8	7	7
44	11	10	11	10	9	9	9	9	8	8
44.5	12	11	12	11	10	10	10	9	9	9
45	12	12	12	11	11	11	10	10	10	10
45.5	13	13	13	12	12	12	11	11	11	10
46	14	14	14	13	13	12	12	12	11	11
46.5	15	14	15	14	13	13	13	12	12	12
47	15	15	15	14	14	14	13	13	13	13
47.5	16	16	16	15	15	15	14	14	14	13
48	17	17	17	16	16	15	15	15	14	14
48.5	18	17	18	17	16	16	16	15	15	15
49	18	18	18	17	17	17	16	16	16	15
49.5	19	19	19	18	18	17	17	17	17	16
50	20	19	20	19	18	18	18	18	17	17
50.5	20	20	20	19	19	19	19	18	18	18
51	21	21	21	20	20	20	19	19	19	18
51.5	22	21	22	21	21	20	20	20	19	19
52	22	22	22	22	21	21	21	20	20	20

Circumference value (in)	TABLE B Women's BF % 2-3 Girth									
	HEIGHT (IN)									
	68	68.5	69	69.5	70	70.5	71	71.5	72	72.5
52.5	23	23	23	22	22	22	21	21	21	20
53	24	23	24	23	23	22	22	22	21	21
53.5	24	24	24	23	23	23	23	22	22	22
54	25	25	25	24	24	24	23	23	23	22
54.5	26	25	26	25	24	24	24	24	23	23
55	26	26	26	25	25	25	24	24	24	24
55.5	27	27	27	26	26	25	25	25	25	24
56	28	27	28	27	26	26	26	25	25	25
56.5	28	28	28	27	27	27	26	26	26	25
57	29	29	29	28	28	27	27	27	26	26
57.5	30	29	29	29	28	28	28	27	27	27
58	30	30	30	29	29	29	28	28	28	27
58.5	31	30	31	30	29	29	29	29	28	28
59	31	31	31	30	30	30	29	29	29	28
59.5	32	32	32	31	31	30	30	30	29	29
60	32	32	32	32	31	31	31	30	30	30
60.5	33	33	33	32	32	31	31	31	31	30
61	34	33	33	33	32	32	32	31	31	31
61.5	34	34	34	33	33	33	32	32	32	31
62	35	34	34	34	34	33	33	33	32	32
62.5	35	35	35	34	34	34	33	33	33	33
63	36	36	35	35	35	34	34	34	33	33
63.5	36	36	36	35	35	35	35	34	34	34
64	37	37	36	36	36	35	35	35	35	34
64.5	38	37	37	37	36	36	36	35	35	35
65	38	38	37	37	37	37	36	36	36	35
65.5	39	38	38	38	37	37	37	36	36	36
66	39	39	39	38	38	38	37	37	37	36
66.5	40	39	39	39	38	38	38	37	37	37
67	40	40	40	39	39	39	38	38	38	37
67.5	41	40	40	40	39	39	39	39	38	38
68	41	41	41	40	40	40	39	39	39	38
68.5	42	41	41	41	40	40	40	40	39	39
69	42	42	42	41	41	41	40	40	40	39
69.5	43	42	42	42	42	41	41	41	40	40
70	43	43	43	42	42	42	41	41	41	40
70.5	44	43	43	43	43	42	42	42	41	41
71	44	44	44	43	43	43	42	42	42	41
71.5	45	44	44	44	43	43	43	43	42	42
72	-	45	45	44	44	44	43	43	43	42
72.5	-	-	-	45	44	44	44	44	43	43
73	-	-	-	-	45	45	44	44	44	43
735.5	-	-	-	-	-	-	45	44	44	44
74	-	-	-	-	-	-	-	45	45	44
74.5	-	-	-	-	-	-	-	-	-	45

TABLE B Women's BF % 2-3 Girth

Circumference value (in)	HEIGHT (IN)									
	73	73.5	74	74.5	75	75.5	76	76.5	77	77.5
34.5-39.5	0	-	-	-	-	-	-	-	-	-
40	1	1	0	0	-	-	-	-	-	-
40.5	2	2	1	1	1	0	0	-	-	-
41	3	2	2	2	2	1	1	1	0	0
41.5	4	3	3	3	2	2	2	2	1	1
42	4	4	4	4	3	3	3	2	2	2
42.5	5	5	5	4	4	4	3	3	3	3
43	6	6	5	5	5	5	4	4	4	3
43.5	7	7	6	6	6	5	5	5	5	4
44	8	7	7	7	6	6	6	6	5	5
44.5	8	8	8	8	7	7	7	6	6	6
45	9	9	9	8	8	8	7	7	7	7
45.5	10	10	9	9	9	9	8	8	8	7
46	11	10	10	10	10	9	9	9	8	8
46.5	12	11	11	11	10	10	10	9	9	9
47	12	12	12	11	11	11	11	10	10	10
47.5	13	13	12	12	12	12	11	11	11	10
48	14	13	13	13	13	12	12	12	11	11
48.5	14	14	14	14	13	13	13	12	12	12
49	15	15	15	14	14	14	13	13	13	13
49.5	16	16	15	15	15	14	14	14	14	13
50	17	16	16	16	15	15	15	15	14	14
50.5	17	17	17	16	16	16	16	15	15	15
51	18	18	17	17	17	17	16	16	16	15
51.5	19	18	18	18	17	17	17	17	16	16
52	19	19	19	18	18	18	18	17	17	17
52.5	20	20	19	19	19	19	18	18	18	17
53	21	20	20	20	20	19	19	19	18	18
53.5	21	21	21	20	20	20	20	19	19	19
54	22	22	21	21	21	21	20	20	20	19
54.5	23	22	22	22	21	21	21	21	20	20
55	23	23	23	22	22	22	22	21	21	21
55.5	24	24	23	23	23	22	22	22	22	21
56	25	24	24	24	23	23	23	22	22	22
56.5	25	25	25	24	24	24	23	23	23	23
57	26	25	25	25	25	24	24	24	23	23
57.5	26	26	26	26	25	25	25	24	24	24
58	27	27	26	26	26	26	25	25	25	24
58.5	28	27	27	27	26	26	26	26	25	25
59	28	28	28	27	27	27	26	26	26	26
59.5	29	28	28	28	28	27	27	27	26	26
60	29	29	29	28	28	28	28	27	27	27
60.5	30	30	29	29	29	28	28	28	28	27
61	31	30	30	30	29	29	29	28	28	28
61.5	31	31	31	30	30	30	29	29	29	28
62	32	31	31	31	30	30	30	30	29	29
62.5	32	32	32	31	31	31	30	30	30	30
63	33	32	32	32	32	31	31	31	30	30
63.5	33	33	33	32	32	32	32	31	31	31
64	34	34	33	33	33	32	32	32	32	31
64.5	34	34	34	34	33	33	33	32	32	32
65	35	35	34	34	34	34	33	33	33	32
65.5	36	35	35	35	34	34	34	33	33	33
66	36	36	35	35	35	35	34	34	34	33
66.5	37	36	36	36	35	35	35	35	34	34
67	37	37	37	36	36	36	35	35	35	34
67.5	38	37	37	37	36	36	36	36	35	35
68	38	38	38	37	37	37	36	36	36	36

Circumference value (in)	HEIGHT (IN)									
	73	73.5	74	74.5	75	75.5	76	76.5	77	77.5
69	39	39	39	38	38	38	37	37	37	37
69.5	40	39	39	39	38	38	38	38	37	37
70	40	40	40	39	39	39	38	38	38	38
70.5	41	40	40	40	39	39	39	39	38	38
71	41	41	41	40	40	40	39	39	39	39
71.5	42	41	41	41	40	40	40	40	39	39
72	42	42	42	41	41	41	40	40	40	40
72.5	43	42	42	42	41	41	41	41	40	40
73	43	43	43	42	42	42	41	41	41	40
73.5	44	43	43	43	42	42	42	42	41	41
74	44	44	43	43	43	43	42	42	42	41
74.5	45	44	44	44	43	43	43	42	42	42
75	-	45	44	44	44	44	43	43	43	42
75.5	-	-	45	45	44	44	44	43	43	42

TABLE B Women's BF % 2-3 Girth

Adapted from Hodgdon and Beckett, 1984.

CLASSIFICATION	% FAT	
	WOMEN	MEN
ESSENTIAL FAT	11.0-14.0	3.0-5.0
LEAN/FIT	15.0-22.0	6.0-15.0
HEALTHY	23.0-26.0	16.0-19.0
RISK	27.0-31.0	20.0-24.0
OBESE	32 and higher	25.0 and higher

PRACTICE EXERCISE 5: SKINFOLD ESTIMATION OF BODY COMPOSITION

Using a workshop participant as a sample subject, perform a skinfold estimation of body fat percentage. Textbook pages 288-290 show the anatomical locations where measurements should be taken.

SKINFOLD CALIPER ESTIMATION OF BODY FAT

Pinching the Skinfold:

1. Locate the correct location using the appropriate landmarks and mark the site of the skinfold with a pen. You may need to wipe the area dry of oils, sweat, or lotions before marking the site.
2. With the thumb and forefingers facing downward, place the fingers perpendicular to the marked site of the skinfold.
3. Using a pinch width of approximately two inches wide, firmly pinch the skinfold between the thumb and first two fingers lifting the subcutaneous fat and skin from the muscle tissue.
4. Place the jaws of the calipers perpendicular to the skinfold site approximately 1 cm below the fingers. The caliper reading should be done approximately halfway between the bottom and top of the fold.
5. Release the trigger of the calipers and read and record the measurement. From the release of the trigger the reading should be done within 2 seconds. Taking a longer period could result in fat compression reducing the true value of the skinfold.

Increasing Test Accuracy:

1. Wait approximately 15 or more seconds before re-measuring a site due to compression of fat.
2. If measurements of any given site varies by more than 1-2 mm, repeat the measurement a third time.
3. If an individual is obese or very muscular, the use of skinfolds may be very difficult. In cases of difficulty leading to inaccuracy the tester may opt to use another applicable type of body composition measurement.
4. Testing experience plays a significant roll in the accuracy of skinfold tests. The more practice and experience gained under an expert instructor the better chance for a true value assessment.
5. Be sure the equipment is properly calibrated before measurements are taken (10 g · mm). Poor instrument selection or incorrect calibration will decrease the accuracy of the reading.

Skinfold Sites – 3 site techniques (see illustrations)

Record results below

Women	Trial #1	Trial #2	Trial #3
1. Tricep	_____ mm	_____ mm	_____ mm
2. Suprailiac	_____ mm	_____ mm	_____ mm
3. Thigh	_____ mm	_____ mm	_____ mm
Sum	_____ mm	_____ mm	_____ mm

Men	Trial #1	Trial #2	Trial #3
1. Chest	_____ mm	_____ mm	_____ mm 8
2. Abdomen	_____ mm	_____ mm	_____ mm 15
3. Thigh	_____ mm	_____ mm	_____ mm
Sum	_____ mm	_____ mm	_____ mm

It is important that the sites chosen for the Skinfold measurement match the charts/formula used for estimation of body fat. The following are illustrations for the sites used for the 3-site technique.

Male Three Sites

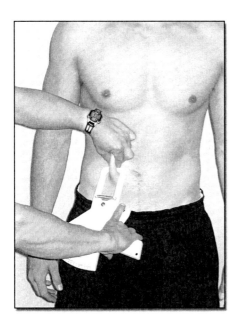

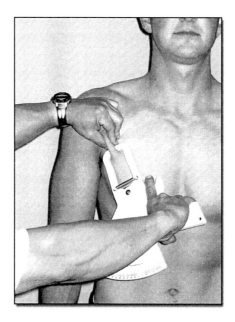

Abdominal Measurement:
Measure a vertical fold 2 cm from the midline of the umbilicus on the right side of the test subject. Be sure that neither the caliper nor the tester's fingers are in the umbilicus during the measurement.

Chest Measurement:
The skinfold is a diagonal fold taken halfway between the anterior axillary line and the nipple. The right side is used for the pinch.

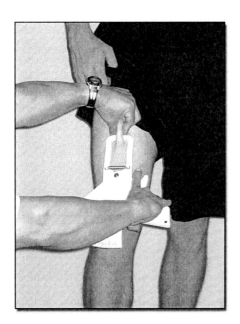

Thigh Measurement:
The measurement is a vertical fold taken over the quadricep muscles on the midline of the right thigh. The measurement should be located halfway between the inguinal crease and the top of the patella.

Female Three Sites

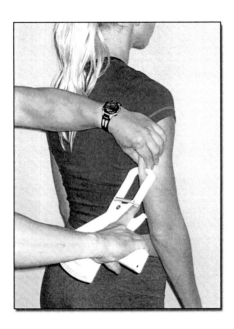

Tricep Measurement:
Measure the vertical fold over the belly of the tricep muscle. Be sure the test subject relaxes the arm. The specific site is located on the posterior midline of the right tricep, halfway between the acromion and olecranon processes.

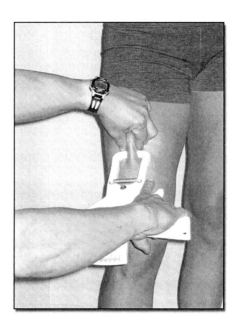

Thigh Measurement:
The measurement is a vertical fold taken over the quadricep muscles on the midline of the right thigh. The measurement should be located halfway between the inguinal crease and the top of the patella.

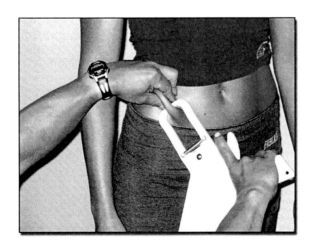

Suprailiac Measurement:
The skinfold is a diagonal fold measured in line with the natural angle of the iliac crest. The measurement should be taken along the anterior axillary line just above the iliac crest on the right side.

If someone is visibly overweight... use girth measurement

Percentage of Body Fat Estimation for *Women* from Age and Triceps, Suprailium, and Thigh Folds								
Sum of skinfolds (mm)	Under 22	23 to 27	28 to 32	33 to 37	38 to 42	43 to 47	48 to 52	53 to 57	Over 57
23-25	9.7	9.9	10.2	10.4	10.7	10.9	11.2	11.4	11.7
26-28	11.0	11.2	11.5	11.7	12.0	12.3	12.5	12.7	13.0
29-31	12.3	12.5	12.8	13.0	13.3	13.5	13.8	14.0	14.3
32-34	13.6	13.8	14.0	14.3	14.5	14.8	15.0	15.3	15.5
35-37	14.8	15.0	15.3	15.5	15.8	16.0	16.3	16.5	16.8
38-40	16.0	16.3	16.5	16.7	17.0	17.2	17.5	17.7	18.0
41-43	17.2	17.4	17.7	17.9	18.2	18.4	18.7	18.9	19.2
44-46	18.3	18.6	18.8	19.1	19.3	19.6	19.8	20.1	20.3
47-49	19.5	19.7	20.0	20.2	20.5	20.7	21.0	21.2	21.5
50-52	20.6	20.8	21.1	21.3	21.6	21.8	22.1	22.3	22.6
53-55	21.7	21.9	22.1	22.4	22.6	22.9	23.1	23.4	23.6
56-58	22.7	23.0	23.2	23.4	23.7	23.9	24.2	24.4	24.7
59-61	23.7	24.0	24.2	24.5	24.7	25.0	25.2	25.5	25.7
62-64	24.7	25.0	25.2	25.5	25.7	26.0	26.2	26.4	26.7
65-67	25.7	25.9	26.2	26.4	26.7	26.9	27.2	27.4	27.7
68-70	26.6	26.9	27.1	27.4	27.6	27.9	28.1	28.4	28.6
71-73	27.5	27.8	28.0	28.3	28.5	28.8	29.0	29.3	29.5
74-76	28.4	28.7	28.9	29.2	29.4	29.7	29.9	30.2	30.4
77-79	29.3	29.5	29.8	30.0	30.3	30.5	30.8	31.0	31.3
80-82	30.1	30.4	30.6	30.9	31.1	31.4	31.6	31.9	32.1
83-85	30.9	31.2	31.4	31.7	31.9	32.2	32.4	32.7	32.9
86-88	31.7	32.0	32.2	32.5	32.7	32.9	33.2	33.4	33.7
89-91	32.5	32.7	33.0	33.2	33.5	33.7	33.9	34.2	34.4
92-94	33.2	33.4	33.7	33.9	34.2	34.4	34.7	34.9	35.2
95-97	33.9	34.1	34.4	34.6	34.9	35.1	35.4	35.6	35.9
98-100	34.6	34.8	35.1	35.3	35.5	35.8	36.0	36.3	36.5
101-103	35.3	35.4	35.7	35.9	36.2	36.4	36.7	36.9	37.2
104-106	35.8	36.1	36.3	36.6	36.8	37.1	37.3	37.5	37.8
107-109	36.4	36.7	36.9	37.1	37.4	37.6	37.9	38.1	38.4
110-112	37.0	37.2	37.5	37.7	38.0	38.2	38.5	38.7	38.9
113-115	37.5	37.8	38.1	38.2	38.5	38.7	39.0	39.2	39.5
116-118	38.0	38.3	38.5	38.8	39.0	39.3	39.5	39.7	40.0
119-121	38.5	38.7	39.0	39.2	39.5	39.7	40.0	40.2	40.5
122-124	39.0	39.2	39.4	39.7	39.9	40.2	40.4	40.7	40.9
125-127	39.4	39.6	39.9	40.1	40.4	40.6	40.9	41.1	41.4
128-130	39.8	40.0	40.3	40.5	40.8	41.0	41.3	41.5	41.8

Percentage of Body Fat Estimation for *Men* from Age and Chest, Abdominal, and Thigh Folds								
Sum of Skinfold (mm)	Under 22	23 to27	28 to 32	33 to 37	38 to 42	43 to 47	48 to 52	53 to 57	Over 57
8-10	1.3	1.8	2.3	2.9	3.4	3.9	4.5	5.0	5.5
11-13	2.2	2.8	3.3	3.9	4.4	4.9	5.5	6.0	6.5
14-16	3.2	3.8	4.3	4.8	5.4	5.9	6.4	7.0	7.5
17-19	4.2	4.7	5.3	5.8	6.3	6.9	7.4	8.0	8.5
20-22	5.1	5.7	6.2	6.8	7.3	7.9	8.4	8.9	9.5
23-25	6.1	6.6	7.2	7.7	8.3	8.8	9.4	9.9	10.5
26-28	7.0	7.6	8.1	8.7	9.2	9.8	10.3	10.9	11.4
29-31	8.0	8.5	9.1	9.6	10.2	10.7	11.3	11.8	12.4
32-34	8.9	9.4	10.0	10.5	11.1	11.6	12.2	12.8	13.3
35-37	9.8	10.4	10.9	11.5	12.0	12.6	13.1	13.7	14.3
38-40	10.7	11.3	11.8	12.4	12.9	13.5	14.1	14.6	15.2
41-43	11.6	12.2	12.7	13.3	13.8	14.4	15.0	15.5	16.1
44-46	12.5	13.1	13.6	14.2	14.7	15.3	15.9	16.4	17.0
47-49	13.4	13.9	14.5	15.1	15.6	16.2	16.8	17.3	17.9
50-52	14.3	14.8	15.4	15.9	16.5	17.1	17.6	18.2	18.8
53-55	15.1	15.7	16.2	16.8	17.4	17.9	18.5	19.1	19.7
56-58	16.0	16.5	17.1	17.7	18.2	18.8	19.4	20.0	20.5
59-61	16.9	17.4	17.9	18.5	19.1	19.7	20.2	20.8	21.4
62-64	17.6	18.2	18.8	19.4	19.9	20.5	21.1	21.7	22.2
65-67	18.5	19.0	19.6	20.2	20.8	21.3	21.9	22.5	23.1
68-70	19.3	19.9	20.4	21.0	21.6	22.2	22.7	23.3	23.9
71-73	20.1	20.7	21.2	21.8	22.4	23.0	23.6	24.1	24.7
74-76	20.9	21.5	22.0	22.6	23.2	23.8	24.4	25.0	25.5
77-79	21.7	22.2	22.8	23.4	24.0	24.6	25.2	25.8	26.3
80-82	22.4	23.0	23.6	24.2	24.8	25.4	25.9	26.5	27.1
83-85	23.2	23.8	24.4	25.0	25.5	26.1	26.7	27.3	27.9
86-88	24.0	24.5	25.1	25.7	26.3	26.9	27.5	28.1	28.7
89-91	24.7	25.3	25.9	26.5	27.1	27.6	28.2	28.8	29.4
92-94	25.4	26.0	26.6	27.2	27.8	28.4	29.0	29.6	30.2
95-97	26.1	26.7	27.3	27.9	28.5	29.1	29.7	30.3	30.9
98-100	26.9	27.4	28.0	28.6	29.2	29.8	30.4	31.0	31.6
101-103	27.5	28.1	28.7	29.3	29.9	30.5	31.1	31.7	32.3
104-106	28.2	28.8	29.4	30.0	30.6	31.2	31.8	32.4	33.0
107-109	28.9	29.5	30.1	30.7	31.3	31.9	32.5	33.1	33.7
110-112	29.6	30.2	30.8	31.4	32.0	32.6	33.2	33.8	34.4
113-115	30.2	30.8	31.4	32.0	32.6	33.2	33.8	34.5	35.1
116-118	30.9	31.5	32.1	32.7	33.3	33.9	34.5	35.1	35.7
119-121	31.5	32.1	32.7	33.3	33.9	34.5	35.1	35.7	36.4

WEIGHT LOSS GOALS – IMPORTANT CONSIDERATIONS

- Current level of body fat (Larger people may lose more weight quickly)
- Current fitness level (Unfit individuals do not have the capacity for hard work)
- Psychology of change (You must want to change)
- Current behaviors (Overeating/drinking and low physical activity obstruct results)
- Reasons for change (Speaks to motivations)
- Lifestyle factors (Time, behaviors)

Learn More: Advanced Concepts of Personal Training Textbook p. 190-193

METABOLIC RATE

Components of Metabolism		
Resting Metabolism (~65%)	Voluntary Metabolism (25-35%) Activity	Thermic Effect of Food (2-10%)

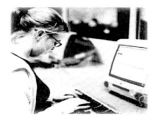
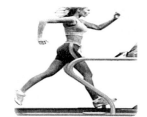
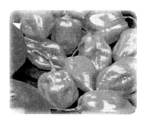

RMR - caloric expenditure needed to sustain physiological processes that typically occur when a person is awake at rest. The primary determinants of RMR are:

1. **Body size**
2. **Muscle mass**
3. **Genetically driven endocrine activity**

Voluntary metabolism – physical activity

Thermic effect of food – energy required to digest and transport nutrients

Learn More: Advanced Concepts of Personal Training Textbook p. 196-197

CALCULATING METABOLIC RATE

- RMR can be calculated using either Lean Mass (Cunningham Formula) or using an individual's gender, age, height, and weight (Modified Harris-Benedict Formula)
- Represents calories needed to maintain current weight at rest

Learn More: Advanced Concepts of Personal Training Textbook p. 196-197

DETERMINING DAILY NEED - TOTAL DAILY ENERGY EXPENDITURE (TDEE)

RMR x {1 + (% of Kcal from thermic effect of food (TEF) + % of Kcal from physical activity PA)} = Daily Need - Total amount of calories expended over the course of the day

Example: 1990 (RMR) x {1 + (5% TEF + 25% PA)} = 1990 x 1.30 = 2587 Kcal

Total Daily Energy Expenditure (TDEE) = 2587 kcal per day

TDEE – RMR = calories from voluntary metabolism
2587 kcal – 1990 kcal = 597 kcals

Learn More: Advanced Concepts of Personal Training Textbook p. 198

INCREASING METABOLISM

- Replace simple sugars and refined carbohydrates with lean protein and plant based foods (whole grains, fruits and vegetables)
- Increase daily physical activity (increase voluntary metabolism)
- Increase the intensity of physical activity (increase EPOC)
- Perform routine resistance training (increase lean mass)

PRACTICAL EXAMPLE

4% increase thermic effect	= -100 kcal/day
1 lb muscle	= -15 kcal/day
High intensity workout (EPOC)	= -65 kcal/day
Net caloric expenditure	= -180 kcal/day
Yearly caloric cost	65,700 kcal (18 lbs fat)

Learn More: Advanced Concepts of Personal Training Textbook p. 197-199

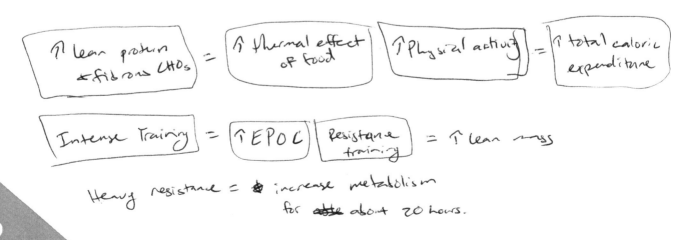

NUTRITION

ENERGY VALUE – MACRONUTRIENTS

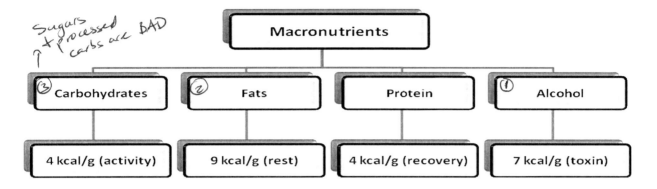

Sugars + processed carbs are BAD?

```
                          Macronutrients
                                 |
        ┌────────────────┬───────────────┬────────────────┐
   ③ Carbohydrates    ② Fats         Protein        ① Alcohol
        |                 |               |                |
 4 kcal/g (activity)  9 kcal/g (rest)  4 kcal/g (recovery)  7 kcal/g (toxin)
```

Learn More: Advanced Concepts of Personal Training Textbook p. 74

CARBOHYDRATES

- Categorized based on length and complexity of the structural chain
- Simple sugars – mono- or disaccharide (glucose, sucrose, fructose, galactose)
- Processed carbohydrates – denatured and simplified – cause problems w/blood glucose
- Starches – polysaccharide (vegetables, grains, cereals, pastas)
- Fiber – cellulose, indigestible except for bacterial breakdown

Learn More: Advanced Concepts of Personal Training Textbook p. 105

EFFECTS OF REFINED SUGARS

- Sucrose/high fructose corn syrup promote dramatic blood sugar spikes
- Increases fat storage potential and reduces fat utilization
- Chronic hyperinsulinemia reduces cellular sensitivity in presence of inflammation
- High consumption increases the risk for obesity and heart disease

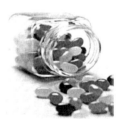

Learn More: Advanced Concepts of Personal Training Textbook p. 107

PROCESSED CARBOHYDRATES

- Manufactured breakdown of grains to a refined product
- Increases glycemic index and potential for lipogenic (fat storage) activity
- Can increase blood triglycerides due to high glycemic loads

Learn More: Advanced Concepts of Personal Training Textbook p. 108

BLOOD GLUCOSE DYNAMICS

- Contributes to the regulation of hunger via the hypothalamus. Without regular small meals hunger becomes appetite and overeating occurs
- Insulin is anabolic and is released in response to the rate and level of blood glucose (glycemic load) which leads to cellular uptake of sugar and hypertrophy of fat cells
- Peaks and valleys in blood glucose levels affect satiety, mood, and caloric intake

Learn More: Advanced Concepts of Personal Training Textbook p. 108-109

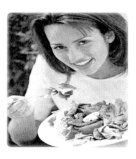

METABOLIC HOMEOSTASIS

- Stable blood glucose (small meals):
  - **Levels blood glucose**
  - **Increases fat utilization**
  - **Reduces risk of fat storage**
  - **Properly regulates hunger**
  - **Can prevent appetite-triggered overeating**
- High glycemic index and load causes greater concentrations of insulin to be produced
- Sustained hyperglycemia causes tissue damage via oxidative stress and metabolic enzyme dysfunction due to glycosylating mechanism

Learn More: Advanced Concepts of Personal Training Textbook p. 107

INADEQUATE CARBOHYDRATES

- Reduction in carbohydrate intake or total calories causes protein catabolism to spare carbohydrates for central nervous system function
- Proteins undergo transamination in muscle, are mobilized into circulation, and deaminated in the liver
- The carbon chains are stripped and converted to glucose (gluconeogenesis)
- Loss of lean mass, metabolic water, and a build up of ketones occurs in a relatively short period of time

Learn More: Advanced Concepts of Personal Training Textbook p. 110

ROLE OF FIBER

Track fiber and water

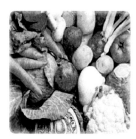

- Type of complex plant carbohydrate (cellulose)
- Cannot be digested by the body
- Provides bulk, aids in food mobility and promotes regular waste elimination which prevents disease and intestinal disorders
- Aids in satiation and can reduce hunger and meal size
- Recommended 20-35 g/day - the average American ingests <15 g/day

Learn More: Advanced Concepts of Personal Training Textbook p. 106

DETERMINING CARBOHYDRATE NEED

$\frac{16}{2.2} = kg$

- US-RDA recommendations; is **55-60% of total diet** be derived from carbohydrates
- Carbohydrates fuel activity; therefore intake is based on activity status
- Sedentary individuals often require lower intakes (45-50%)

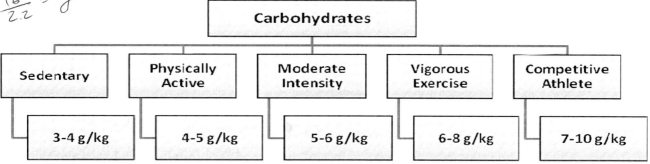

Source: Sports Science Exchange

Learn More: Advanced Concepts of Personal Training Textbook p. 112

POST-EXERCISE REPLENISHMENT

3 carbs : 1 protein   up to 60g. of carbs.

- 3:1 Carbohydrate to Protein mix (chocolate milk)
- Up to 60g CHO/20g Protein causes hypersaturation of glycogen; promote protein synthesis
- Competitive training requires total work calories replaced within 4-5 hours

ROLE OF PROTEIN

- Contributes to 5-15% of total daily energy
- Function - build and repair tissue and structures of the body
- Intake should be **~10-15% of diet**, increase for weight loss/diabetes

Learn More: Advanced Concepts of Personal Training Textbook p. 117

PROTEIN CONSIDERATIONS

- 20 different amino acids required by the body - 8 are essential
- Complete proteins contain all eight essential amino acids
- Daily requirements are dependent on physical activity requirements of the body

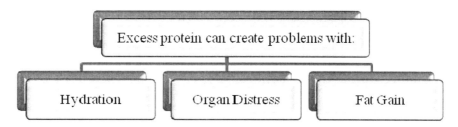

Learn More: Advanced Concepts of Personal Training Textbook p. 118

DETERMINING NEED

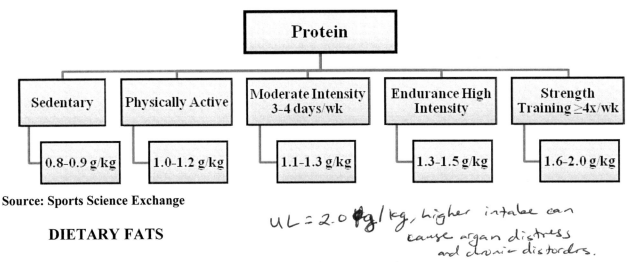

Source: **Sports Science Exchange**

DIETARY FATS

UL = 2.0 øg/kg, higher intake can cause organ distress and chronic disorders.

Differ in chain length and degree of hydrogen saturation
  Saturated Fatty Acids *gets converted in liver, ↑LDL cholesterol.*
    Single bonded straight chain
    Recommended intake <10% of diet
    Ingesting saturated fats elevates bad blood cholesterol (LDL-C)
Unsaturated Fatty Acids
    Missing hydrogen(s) in fatty acid chain and contain double bonds
    Monounsaturated fat is cardiovascularly benign (Mediterranean Diet)
Polyunsaturated: Omega-3 PUFAs *—nuts and cold water fish*
    Shown to be cardioprotective by increasing arachidonic acid which is a precursor to
    hormones involved in vasodilaiton and improved blood flow. They also are associated
    with antioxidant actions that reduce atherosclerotic processes and risk of CAD.
Trans Fatty Acids *- Ø at all!! "Partially hydrogenated veg. oil"*
    Hydrogenated cis-fatty acids become trans fatty acids
    Used to change the texture/composition of food materials
    Recommended <1% of the diet
    Increase LDL-C and reduce HDL-C increasing CAD risk more dramatically than
    saturated fatty acids
Monounsaturated should be the most.
    Learn More: Advanced Concepts of Personal Training Textbook p. 112-114

DETERMINING NEED

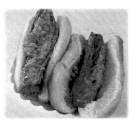

- Fat represents a large fuel source – 9 calories per gram
- Aerobic exercise reduces blood triglycerides and increases HDL-C

General Recommendations:
- <20% requires a physician approval
- 20-25% for weight loss or risk for CAD
- **25-30% of calories from dietary fat is recommended for healthy adults**
- 35% for extreme caloric expenditure such as endurance athletes

    Learn More: Advanced Concepts of Personal Training Textbook p. 113

ANTIOXIDANTS

too many antioxidants will block ability to ↑ muscle

- β-carotene (vitamin A precursor), vitamin A, vitamin C, vitamin E
- Neutralize free-radicals formed from oxygen molecules (2-5% of oxygen)
- Vitamin C should be increased for smokers and high volume activity
- Excess intake may inhibit adaptation response

Learn More: Advanced Concepts of Personal Training Textbook p. 124

NUTRIENT DEFICIENCIES

Calcium

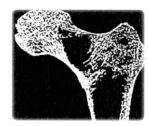

- Crucial for maintenance of strong bones and teeth
- Insufficient levels cause calcium to be drawn from bone leading to decreased density and possible osteoporosis
- **RDA - 1300 mg/day to age 18 and 1000 mg/day thereafter**
- Increased need for pregnant and postmenopausal women
- American women on average consume less than 500-700 mg/day

Iron

Iron + Vit C = triple iron

- Iron-deficiency is the most common nutritional deficiency among child-bearing age women, infants, young children, and adolescents (also among endurance athletes)
- **Requirements are 8-10 mg/day for men and postmenopausal women**
- **18 mg/day for women during child-bearing years**
- Iron absorption is tripled if consumed with vitamin C

Learn More: Advanced Concepts of Personal Training Textbook p. 127-129

ELECTROLYTES

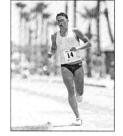

- Sodium, chloride, potassium, and magnesium
- Renal/hormonal regulation of electrolytes is crucial to cellular function
- Sodium/potassium are regulated by aldosterone for cellular fluid balance
- Training in heat results in extracellular fluid loss which reduces blood plasma and disrupts intra/extra cellular fluid balance

Learn More: Advanced Concepts of Personal Training Textbook p. 130

EFFECTS OF DEHYDRATION

- Water intake should reflect activity and environment exposure
- 8-10 ounces (250 ml) every 10-15 minutes during exercise
- Sweat rate, electrolyte balance, temperature, altitude, and beginning fluid balance will determine additional water intake needs
- Exercise in the heat often requires a carb-electrolyte solution of 4-8%
- Effects of dehydration:
  - 1-2% decrease in total body volume = **2-5% decrease in performance**
  - 3% decrease in total body volume = **8-10% decrease in performance**
  - 5% decrease in total body volume = **High risk for heat illness**

Learn More: Advanced Concepts of Personal Training Textbook p. 130-136

1200 mg Calcium to optimize fat burning.

BIOMECHANICS – TERM REVIEW AND APPLICATION

ANATOMICAL POSITION TERMS

- Anterior
- Posterior
- Inferior
- Superior
- Proximal
- Distal
- Lateral
- Medial
- Supine
- Prone

Learn More: Advanced Concepts of Personal Training Textbook p. 9-10

PLANES OF MOVEMENT

- Sagittal
- Transverse
- Frontal

Learn More: Advanced Concepts of Personal Training Textbook p. 8

MUSCLE FUNCTION DESCRIPTORS

- Agonist
- Antagonist
- Prime mover
- Neutralizer
- Stabilizer
- Accelerator
- Decelerator

Learn More: Advanced Concepts of Personal Training Textbook p. 40-42

CONTRACTIONS

- Concentric
- Eccentric
- Isometric
- Isokinetic
- Isotonic
- Static
- Dynamic
- Ballistic

Learn More: Advanced Concepts of Personal Training Textbook p. 57

JOINT MOVEMENTS - VERTEBRAL COLUMN

- Cervical Vertebra – C1-C7
- Thoracic Vertebra – T1-T12
- Lumbar Vertebra – L1-L5
- Sacrum

ACTIONS	PRIME MOVER	EXERCISE
Flexion	Rectus abdominis	Ab-curl up
Extension	Erector spinae	Back extension
Rotation	Obliques	Cable torso twist
Lateral Flexion	Obliques/Quadratus lumborum	Oblique crunch
Stability	Transverse abdominis	Draw-in techniques

Learn More: Advanced Concepts of Personal Training Textbook p. 15-17

GLENOHUMERAL JOINT

ACTIONS	PRIME MOVER	EXERCISE
Flexion	Anterior Deltoid	Front raise
Extension	Latissimus dorsi	Pullover
Hyperextension	Rhomboids	Seated row
Adduction	Latissimus dorsi	Pull-up
Abduction	Deltoid	Side raise
Horizontal Abduction	Posterior Deltoid	Rear delt pull
Horizontal Adduction	Pectoralis major	Bench press
Internal Rotation	Subscapularis	Band rotation
External Rotation	Teres minor/infraspinatus	Hitchhikers

Learn More: Advanced Concepts of Personal Training Textbook p. 18-20

SHOULDER COMPLEX

ACTIONS	PRIME MOVER	EXERCISE
Elevation	Trapezius	Shrugs
Depression	Pec minor/Trap/Levator scapulae	Scapula dips
Retraction	Rhomboids	Seated row
Protraction	Pec minor/Serratus anterior	Single Arm Reach

Learn More: Advanced Concepts of Personal Training Textbook p. 21-22

PELVIS

ACTIONS	PRIME MOVER	EXERCISE
Anterior Tilt	Iliopsoas/Erector spinae	Pelvic Bridging
Posterior Tilt	Rectus abdominis	Abdominal curl-up

Learn More: Advanced Concepts of Personal Training Textbook p. 18

HIP

ACTIONS	PRIME MOVER	EXERCISE
Flexion	Iliopsoas	Knee raise
Extension	Gluteus maximus	Squat
Abduction	Tensor fascia latae	Lateral lunge
Adduction	Gracilis/Adductor longus	Lateral step up
Internal Rotation	Glute min/medius	Transverse lunge
External Rotation	Piriformis/Quad femoris	Transverse step down

Learn More: Advanced Concepts of Personal Training Textbook p. 24

KNEE

ACTIONS	PRIME MOVER	EXERCISE
Flexion	Bicep femoris Semitendinosus Semimembranosus	Leg curl
Extension	Rectus femoris Vastus lateralis Vastus intermedius Vastus medialis	Leg extension

Learn More: Advanced Concepts of Personal Training Textbook p. 25-26

ANKLE

ACTIONS	PRIME MOVER	EXERCISE
Plantar flexion	Gastroc/Soleus	Heel raise
Dorsi flexion	Anterior tibialis	Toe raise

Learn More: Advanced Concepts of Personal Training Textbook p. 27

ENERGY TRANSFER TERMS

Kinetic chain – energy transferred through the body through force couples

Ground reaction forces – initiation of energy transfer often beginning with ground based contractile force application commonly seen in closed chain activities

Open vs. closed chain – distal contact position; closed chain suggests all aspects of the anatomical chain are closed and distally fixed as seen in a squat; open chain suggests the chain has an open component as seen in the leg curl/extension where the feet contribute no reaction force

Learn More: Advanced Concepts of Personal Training Textbook p. 471

TRUNK TRAINING

Base Movement	Progression One	Progression Two
Draw-in technique		
Draw-in and Ab curl-up	Ab curl-up w/targeting	Ab curl-up w/torque
Reverse crunch	- w/curl-up	- w/ OH reach or jackknife
Opposite raise	Quadruped (w/assessment)	
Prone plank (assessment)	- w/hip extension	Athlete's plank
Supine pelvic bridge	- w/balance	- SL and balance
Supine bench bridge	- w/marching (legs only)	- w/alternate arm/leg march
Trunk stabilization (bench)	- add OH reach	- add alternating marches
Good morning	- w/elbow reach	- w/ITY reaches and/or SL
Split stance rotation	- w/step	- w/alternate marches
Standing neutral rotation	Diagonal chop	SL diagonal chop w/ flexion

FLEXIBILITY ASSESSMENT

The NCSF has incorporated the use of eleven field flexibility assessments for multi-joint evaluation of ROM. Due to the fact that flexibility is a joint specific trait, assessing only one or two separate areas will not give you an accurate representation of a subject's overall flexibility. The tests outlined below focus on four primary areas, where over twenty different muscle groups are assessed in the eleven field tests. **The benefits of these tests include joint-specific ROM analysis, ease of execution, limited equipment use, and immediate feedback.**

Shoulder
- Shoulder Flexion
- Shoulder Abduction
- Shoulder Rotators

Trunk
- Trunk Flexion
- Trunk Extension
- Trunk Lateral Flexion
- Trunk Rotation

Hip
- Hip Flexion
- Hip Extension

Leg
- Knee Flexion
- Knee Extension

TYPES OF FLEXIBILITY TRAINING

Static
Active
Active-Assisted
Active-Isolation
PNF

Passive
Assisted Range of Motion

Dynamic
Movements through full ROM
Multi-planar full ROM

Learn More: Advanced Concepts of Personal Training Textbook p. 339-343

Exercise Prescription for Flexibility Overview

Assessing Flexibility	Goniometer, Measurements Movement Screens Field Tests	One test cannot measure or identify total flexibility or ROM limitations
Frequency of Training	Minimum 2-3 x/week	Stretching can be performed everyday
Volume of training	Ideal duration of each static stretch is 30-45 seconds	Each body part should be stretched twice a week
Types of Training	Static, Dynamic, PNF, and Partner assisted *Ballistic stretching can cause injury*	Make selections based on expertise, goals, time, and ROM capabilities
Components of Flexibility	Decrease resistance from the agonist muscle and increase the strength of the antagonist Increased in sarcomeres along myofibril Increase tendon length	Flexibility training attempts to elicit a plastic response from the muscle fascia Elastic response is a temporary adjustment Plastic response is an adaptation
Physiological Adaptations	Increased Tissue Relaxation Increased Tissue Elongation Increased Tissue Pliability	Affected Tissue and Structures: Muscle, Fascia, Tendons, Nerves, Blood Vessels

Joint Movers	Category	Muscle Group	Stretch
Plantar Flexors	Active Isolation	Gastrocnemius	AI dorsi flexion
Knee Flexors	Active Isolation	Hamstrings	AI leg extension
Hip Extensors	Active Isolation	Gluteus max/med	AI hip flexion
Hip Abductors	Active	TFL, Glute min/med	Active cross over
Knee Extensors	Active Isolation	Quadriceps	AI leg flexion
Hip Flexors	Dynamic	Iliopsoas	Active lunge w/reach
Hip Adductors	Active	Long adductors	Active side lunge
Hip External Rotator	Dynamic	Piriformis	Active hip flexion
Shoulder H. Adductors	Active Assisted	Pectoralis major	Unilateral T-stretch
Shoulder Extensors	Active Isolation	Latissimus dorsi	AI shoulder abduction
Shoulder Flexors	Active Assisted	Anterior deltoid	Active back arm cross
Shoulder Rotators	Active Assisted	Int/ext rotators	AI shoulder rotators

AEROBIC EXERCISE PRESCRIPTION

GOALS OF AEROBIC TRAINING

- 10-30% increase in VO_2max via cardiac and muscular augmentation
  - ✓ **Increases lifespan**
- Improved vascular compliance enhances endothelial function and vascular wall pliability
  - ✓ **Reduces CAD**
- Mediation of inflammatory chemicals reduces risk for disease
  - ✓ **Hypertension, hyperlipidemia, diabetes**
- Stimulates parasympathetic action reducing blood pressure
  - ✓ **Lowers blood pressure and heart stress**
- Improved heart efficiency reduces heart rate and stress
  - ✓ **Improves QOL**

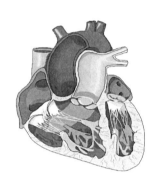

Ability to use Oxygen:

- Correlates to life expectancy
- Affects risk for disease
- Affects anaerobic and aerobic performance outcomes
- Affects caloric expenditure
- Affects quality of life

Learn More: Advanced Concepts of Personal Training Textbook p. 363

CARDIAC OUTPUT

cardiac output

- CO = SV x HR represents the volume of blood expelled by the heart per minute
- After training effect, the HR is lower at a given oxygen demand due to greater SV
- The increase in SV with training accompanies an increase in tissue oxygen utilization

HEART RATE
- Number of times blood is expelled from the heart in one minute
- At about 110 bpm the heart rate increases linearly with work
- Predicted Max HR = 220 - age (+ or -) up to 3 standard deviations of 10-12 bpm
- Higher VO_2 max = lower HR at any given intensity except maximal efforts

STROKE VOLUME (SV)
- The blood pumped from the heart per beat (expelled from left ventricle)
- Endurance-trained hearts expel more blood per beat
- SV increases then levels off at about 40% VO_2 max
- After 40% VO_2max, increases in HR are solely responsible for meeting output demands
- Higher resting SV seen with endurance training accounts for lower HR at rest
- Endurance training increases ventricular volume

Learn More: Advanced Concepts of Personal Training Textbook p. 93

systolic

HR x SBP = Rate - Pressure Product (RPP)

RATE PRESSURE PRODUCT

- Heart Rate x Systolic Blood Pressure = RPP
- Oxygen demands of the heart (stress)
- Makes exercise harder for new clients due to:
  - Increased sympathetic response (heart work)
  - Increased oxygen demand
  - Hyperventilation (diaphragm work)
- Lower BP and RHR reduce perceived and actual exertion

Learn More: Advanced Concepts of Personal Training Textbook p. 102

AEROBIC TRAINING ADAPTATIONS

$$VO_2 = CARDIAC\ OUTPUT\ X\ (A\text{-}V)\ O_2\ DIFFERENCE$$

Heart

Myocardial adaptations to improve O_2 delivery	Muscular adaptations to improve O_2 extraction
• Increased stroke volume ↑ • Improved conduction efficiency • Increased metabolic efficiency • Reduced HR at all sub-maximal levels	• Increased capillary density • Increased mitochondria • Increased aerobic (oxidative) enzyme concentrations *—ability to hold O_2 in muscle cell* • Increased myoglobin and lactate threshold • Asynchronous firing patterns

→ during cardio, muscle fibers fire seperately (take turns) (Weight lifting is synchronized)

- These adaptations increase tissue O_2 consumption, measured by difference in arterial O_2 content (from the heart and lungs) from venous O_2 content (back to the heart and lungs)
- This measurement is the (a-v) O_2 difference

Learn More: Advanced Concepts of Personal Training Textbook p. 93-95

SKELETAL MUSCLE ADAPTATIONS

INCREASED OXIDATIVE PATHWAYS THROUGH:
- Enzyme concentration shifts toward aerobic metabolism
- Increased mitochondria density in trained cells
- Increased capillaries to working tissues
- Fast twitch glycolytic fibers shift to fast twitch oxidative/glycolytic fibers
- Type I fibers become more efficient metabolically

Learn More: Advanced Concepts of Personal Training Textbook p. 60

Cardio exercises will increase muscle endurance and mitochondrial production.

☆ How long does it take to increase mitochondria?

TRAINING ZONES

HEART RATE MAX METHOD
- 220 - age x Training Intensity
- Assumes all people of the same age should train at the same level
- Training range 75-90% (Max HR)

HEART RATE RESERVE METHOD
- HRR = Max HR - Resting HR (the range is individual specific)
- Karvonen Formula = HRR x (training intensity) + RHR
- Factors in stroke volume
- Training range used in the formula 60-80%

Heart Rate Target

Age	55%	60%	70%	80%	85%
15	19	21	24	27	29
20	18	20	23	27	28
25	18	19	23	26	28
30	17	19	22	25	27
35	17	19	22	25	26
40	17	18	21	24	26
45	16	18	20	23	25
50	16	17	20	23	24
55	15	17	19	22	23
60	15	16	19	21	23
65	14	16	18	21	22
70	14	15	18	20	21
75	13	15	17	19	21
80	13	14	16	19	20

Learn More: Advanced Concepts of Personal Training Textbook p. 355-357

HEART RATE MAX FORMULA

Max HR is 220 - age (SD = +/- 10-12 beats)
Prediction is reduced for ages <15 or >60

Example for a 20-year-old
220 - 20 years = 200 BPM

Learn More: Advanced Concepts of Personal Training Textbook p. 355

HEART RATE RESERVE (KARVONEN FORMULA)

FORMULATION OF THE EXERCISE PRESCRIPTION

- Program intensities are based on Target HR zones and RPE
- Training thresholds for fit populations are 60-80% of VO₂max and HRR Method (Karvonen)

HEART RATE RESERVE (HRR) EQUATION

Heart Rate Reserve = Max HR – Resting HR
Example 20-year-old with a RHR of 60 BPM
220 – 20 years = 200 BPM
200 – 60 = 140 BPM (HRR)

KARVONEN METHOD (60-80% INTENSITY RANGE)
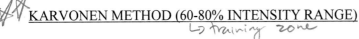
↳ training zone

Heart Rate Reserve = (Max HR – Resting HR) x intensity + RHR

Example for a 20 year-old with a resting HR of 60 BPM
220 – 20 years = 200 BPM
200 – 60 = 140 BPM
140 x .60 = 84 + 60 = 144 BPM
140 x .80 = 112 + 60 = 172 BPM

Learn More: Advanced Concepts of Personal Training Textbook p. 357

@ 60% → hydrogen build up
@ 80% → hydrogen dumped into blood

208 – (.7 x age)

PRACTICE EXERCISE 6: CALCULATING AEROBIC TRAINING INTENSITIES

Cardiovascular Training Intensities

Resting Heart Rate (RHR): 75 BPM (60 seconds)

Age: 40

20 (handwritten)

Calculate Max Heart Rate

220 – __*20*__ age = __*200*__ Max Heart Rate

40 (handwritten)

220 – 40 = 180 MHR

180 – 75 = 105 HRR

Calculate Heart Rate Reserve

__*200*__ Max Heart Rate – __*60*__ Resting Heart Rate = __*140*__ Heart Rate Reserve (HRR)

105 HRR × 60% = 63 + 75 = 138 Low HR

105 × .8 = 84 + 75 = 159 high HR

Calculate Training Zone using the Karvonen Formula

(__*140*__ HRR x 60%) = __*84*__ BPM + __*60*__ RHR = __*144*__ Low-end HR range

(__*140*__ HRR x 80%) = __*172*__ BPM + __*60*__ RHR = __*172*__ High-end HR range

Training Zones: Low-end range __*144*__ BPM to High-end range __*172*__ BPM

Trainig Zones: 138 – 159 HR (handwritten)

RATE OF PERCEIVED EXERTION (BORG SCALE)

- Represents individual/subjective perceived exertion of participant
- The 6-20 scale equates to 60-200 BPM
- Using RPE 12-14 = 60-80% VO$_2$max or Karvonen formula
- Cardiac patients may use RPE solely for exercise
- **Talk Test:** when the client finds it difficult to speak about 3 sentences in a row, or they can hear their own breathing – they are close to their ventilatory threshold

1 – 10 = easy
12 – 14 = training zone
15 – 20 = hard (should be able to say 3 sentences in a row. More then that is too hard)

TRAINING INTENSITIES

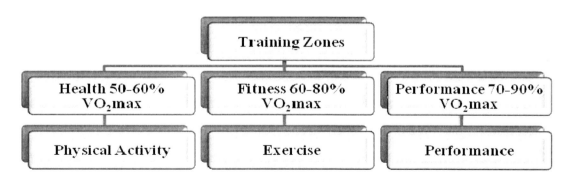

- Moderate intensities are associated with optimal health and lifespan – harder is not better as the stress outweighs the benefits
- Higher intensities yield elevated caloric expenditure during and after exercise

For marathon training = ↓60% more than ↑80%

47

ENERGY SOURCE CONTRIBUTION

- **Fats** - highest percentage at low intensities/rest (≈70% at rest)
- **Glycogen** - increases with intensity; primary fuel for higher intensity work; is used aerobically and anaerobically
- **Protein** - used sparingly unless hypoglycemic, undernourished, or carbohydrate depleted

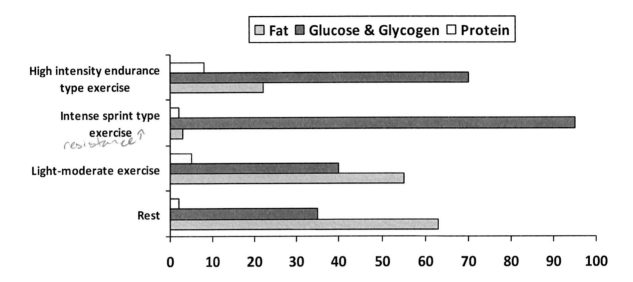

Learn More: Advanced Concepts of Personal Training Textbook p. 358

Lifting weights enhances metabolism

FAT BURNING ZONE VS. HIGH INTENSITY

- Sleep and rest are optimal fat-burning zone activities
- Low intensity training = low caloric expenditure
- High intensity training burns more fat and calories during the same time period
- High intensity = longer EPOC stimulating adrenal hormones to increase fat use in recovery

Learn More: Advanced Concepts of Personal Training Textbook p. 358

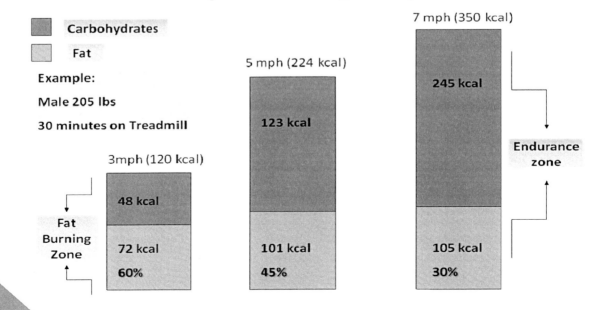

INTERVAL TRAINING VS. STEADY STATE

STEADY STATE TRAINING
- No change in heart rate over five (5) BPM
- Generally used for acclimation or longer duration training bouts

INTERVAL TRAINING
- Varied intensity for higher work rates
- Higher excess post-exercise oxygen consumption (EPOC) and caloric yield
- Faster rate of aerobic adaptations

Learn More: Advanced Concepts of Personal Training Textbook p. 357

CALORIC PITFALLS

- Machine calculations of calories are based on METS and defined variables which may not be correct (elliptical trainer)

[handwritten: └→ over-predicts by ~30%   ONLY look at HR]

```
┌────────────────────────────────────────────────────────────┐
│   Behaviors that ↓ expenditure below displayed value         │
└────────────────────────────────────────────────────────────┘
┌──────────────────┐  ┌──────────────────┐  ┌──────────────────┐
│ Leaning on a     │  │ Holding onto     │  │ Failing to       │
│ weight bearing   │  │ guiderails       │  │ complying with   │
│ machine          │  │                  │  │ default RPMs     │
└──────────────────┘  └──────────────────┘  └──────────────────┘
```

[handwritten: Sprinting will train cardiac abilities without affecting muscles]

CONCURRENT HIGH INTENSITY TRAINING

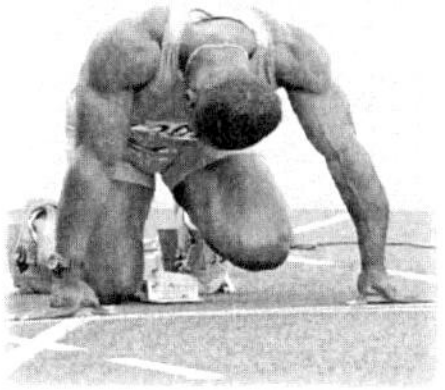

ANAEROBIC
- Increase neuromuscular efficiency
- Increase lactate threshold
- Increase power output

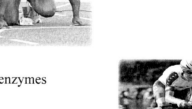

AEROBIC
- Decrease anaerobic enzymes with increased aerobic enzymes
- Decrease in size and power output of type II fibers
- Increase mitochondrial and capillary density
- Conversion of type IIb to type IIa muscle fibers

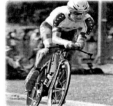

Learn More: Advanced Concepts of Personal Training Textbook p. 389-390

[handwritten: What do I do about detraining effect? └→ periods of training volume decline? INCREASE intensity]

CARDIOVASCULAR DETRAINING EFFECT

- Within 12 days VO$_2$max decreases by 7% with training cessation
- Primary acute response – decreased CO (SV)
- Reduced training or cessation also causes decrease max O$_2$ extraction
- Prevented or reduced by increasing the training intensity even with shorter durations

Learn More: Advanced Concepts of Personal Training Textbook p. 365

ANAEROBIC TRAINING

ANAEROBIC TRAINING GOALS

Potential benefits
•Neuromuscular coordination – enhance movement proficiency •Strength balance – maintain joint health and function •Increased force production – improve strength •Muscle hypertrophy – increase size and metabolic fitness •Increased power – increase rate of acceleration •Local muscular endurance – improve ability to sustain activity/stability •Improved range of motion – improve ability to move, musculoskeletal enhancements •Metabolic enhancements – increase rate and energy system efficiency •Increased bone density – strengthen bones •Enhanced movement confidence – increase physical activity •Improved quality of life

Learn More: Advanced Concepts of Personal Training Textbook p. 371

ANAEROBIC ENERGY SYSTEMS

- Immediate (phosphagen) – nervous system training
  - ATP splits into ADP + Pi = 1RM (3 seconds)
    - **~90 seconds recovery**
  - CP splits, energy rephosphorylates ATP = 3RM (10-15 seconds)
    - *creatine phosphate* **2-5 minutes recovery**
- Intermediate (CHOs) – muscular system training
  - Glycogen through glycolysis = up to 90 seconds of work
    - **30-90 seconds recovery**

FIBER CONTRIBUTION

- **Type II B/X (FTG)**
  Anaerobic – Large diameter
  50 grams of force per motor unit/5 minute fatigue rate
- **Type II A (FTG/O)**
  Anaerobic/Aerobic – Medium diameter
  30 grams of force/6 minute fatigue rate
- **Type I (STO)**
  Aerobic – Small diameter
  5 grams of force/fatigue resistant

Heavy loads recruit all 3 fibers
High velocity recruits fast twitch.
Low velocity low weights recruits slower twitch fibers

MAXIMAL STRENGTH

[handwritten: low rep power First, low prep strength 2nd moderate rep 3rd→hyper. anarobic cap. 4rth aerobic cap. 5th.]

KEY FACTORS

- Neuromuscular efficiency
- Neural overload
- Adequate rest intervals for phosphagen energy replenishment
- Stabilizers are often the weak link

TRAINING GUIDELINES

- Intensity: 75-95% 1RM   Phosphagen (87.5%-95%) Glycolytic (75-85%)
- Frequency: 3-5x/week
- Volume: Low (18-30 scts/day)
- Mode: Cross joint lifts *[handwritten: nervous system   muscle]*
- Repetitions: 3-5 (phosphagen) 6-10 (glycolytic)
- Rest Interval: 60-90 sec (glycolytic) 2-5 minutes (phosphagen)
- Emphasis: Force production (neural efficiency)
- Endocrine response: GH and testosterone
- Systems: Pyramid sets, Negative sets

Learn More: Advanced Concepts of Personal Training Textbook p. 382-385

[handwritten: W/heavy weight → ↑ release of testosterone]

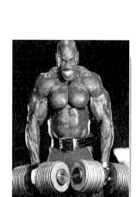

HYPERTROPHY

KEY FACTORS

- Anabolic hormone concentration (physiological disruption)
- Fiber recruitment – number and type
- Application and amount of overload (high volume, prolonged overload)
- Adequate recovery and nutritional support

TRAINING GUIDELINES   *[handwritten: FAST FAST FAST]*

- Intensity: 70-85% 1RM
- Frequency: 4-6x/week
- Volume: High (30-40 sets/day)
- Mode: Isolated Lifts
- Repetitions: 8-12 (8-10 high anabolic)
- Rest Interval: 30-60 seconds (up to 90 sec. on heaviest lifts)
- Emphasis: Muscle Fiber Recruitment
- Endocrine response: testosterone, GH, cortisol, epinephrine and **IGF-1**
- Systems: Complexes, Supersets, Strip sets

Learn More: Advanced Concepts of Personal Training Textbook p. 381-382

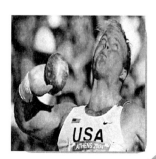

MUSCULAR POWER

KEY FACTORS

- Speed of movement – velocity specific
- Inverse relationship between force and velocity
- Pre-load enhances neural contribution

TRAINING GUIDELINES

- Intensity: 30-50% 1RM (glycolytic) or 60-95% 1RM (CP)

[handwritten: Olympic lifts]

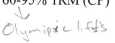

- Frequency: 2-4x/week
- Volume: Varied by activity (Moderate)
- Mode: Olympic lifts, ballistics, plyometrics
- Repetitions: Vary by activity speed/intensity/energy system; 2-5 (CP), 8-20 (Glycolytic)
- Rest interval: 30-240 seconds(depending on power rate)
- Emphasis: Movement Speed
- Endocrine response: GH, testosterone and epinephrine
- Systems: Plyometrics, Contrast sets

Learn More: Advanced Concepts of Personal Training Textbook p. 385-386

ANAEROBIC ENDURANCE

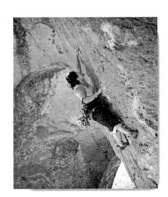

KEY FACTORS
- Muscle strength (reduces intensity of submaximal work)
- Fiber recruitment patterns
- Cellular energy efficiency
- By-product removal capabilities (buffering)

TRAINING GUIDELINES
- Intensity: 50-70% 1RM
- Frequency: 3-5x/week
- Volume: 30-45 sets/day
- Mode: Multiple modality
- Repetitions: 12-25
- Rest interval: 20-30 seconds
- Emphasis: Cellular Energy Efficiency
- Endocrine response: minimal GH and epinephrine
- Systems: Supersets, Circuits

Learn More: Advanced Concepts of Personal Training Textbook p. 386-388

GENERAL FITNESS

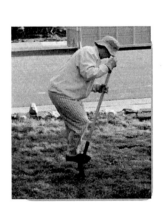

KEY FACTORS
- Load assignment/bone stress (compound exercises preferred)
- Weight bearing over non-weight bearing
- Coordinated movements
- Full ROM

TRAINING GUIDELINES
- Intensity: 50-75% 1RM
- Frequency: 3-5x/week
- Volume: 30-36 sets/day
- Mode: Mutli-planer movements, Multiple modality
- Repetitions: 8-20
- Rest interval: 30-60 seconds
- Emphasis: Improved Health and Fitness
- Endocrine response: limited GH, testosterone, and adrenals
- Systems Combinations, Supersets, Circuits

Learn More: Advanced Concepts of Personal Training Textbook p. 388-389

GOALS OF TRAINING

- Training parameters must shift to reflect the principle of specificity
- Training prescription must match the desired adaptation response by specific demand (overload)
- Force production is stability and velocity limited

INTENSITY BY REPETITION

1RM – 100%	4RM – 90%	7RM – 82.5%	10RM – 75%
2RM – 95%	5RM – 87.5%	8RM – 80%	11RM – 72.5%
3RM – 92.5%	6RM – 85%	9RM – 77.5%	12RM – 70%

- Over 12 repetitions predictions vary due to strength : stability relationship

Learn More: Advanced Concepts of Personal Training Textbook p. 410

METHODS OF TRAINING

[handwritten: hard exercise 1st]   *[handwritten: same muscle]*

- Superset – two or three exercises (tri-set) in a row with no rest interval *[handwritten: back squat then jumping]*
- Contrast Set – superset using a heavy slow set combined with a light fast set
- Strip Set – same exercise repeated without rest using decreasing loads
- Combination Exercise – two exercises fused to form one *[handwritten: large w/rotation -> not large then rotation]*
- Pyramid Training – technique based on neural preparation to heavier loads – *[handwritten: strength]* *[handwritten: reduce reps increase weight %]*
- Negative Training – greater than 1RM load used during eccentric movement *[handwritten: pushing back]*
- Circuit Training – grouping of exercises performed in sequence
- Complex Training – exercises grouped by muscle or joint

Learn More: Advanced Concepts of Personal Training Textbook p. 377-380

PRACTICE EXERCISE 7: USING TRAINING SYSTEMS

Combination Exercise   *[handwritten: step up w/curl ;]*

Hypertrophy Superset   *[handwritten: Bench press]* + *[handwritten: lat pulldown]*

Contrast Set   *[handwritten: snatch w/little bls]* + *[handwritten: squat jumps]*

Pyramid Training using (130 lb 1RM)

10RM 100 lbs.   8RM *[handwritten: 105]* lbs.   6RM *[handwritten: 110]* lbs.

[handwritten: b: 80% = 130 x .8 = 105]

Learn More: Advanced Concepts of Personal Training Textbook p. 377-380

[handwritten: 9 rep w/weight -> input -> tells you how much weight]

EXERCISE CONSIDERATIONS

- What is the purpose of this exercise?
- Does this exercise promote the desired outcome response?
- Is this exercise appropriate for this individual and at this point in the training cycle?
- Does this exercise complement other training factors?
- Does it fit in the training program?

Learn More: Advanced Concepts of Personal Training Textbook p. 314

EXERCISE SELECTION

Hypertrophy	Strength	Power	Function
Seated dumbbell press	Military press	Push press	Unilateral cable press
Smith machine lunge	Barbell lunge	Jump lunges	Lunges with rotation
Adductor machine	Lateral squats	Lateral step rebounds	MB overhead lateral lunge

EXERCISE ORDER CRITERIA

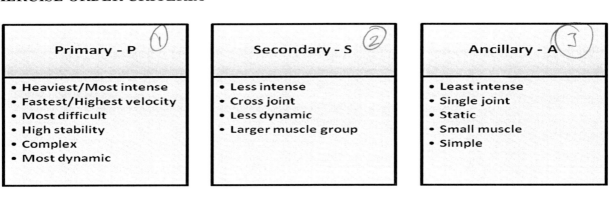

Primary - P ①	Secondary - S ②	Ancillary - A ③
• Heaviest/Most intense • Fastest/Highest velocity • Most difficult • High stability • Complex • Most dynamic	• Less intense • Cross joint • Less dynamic • Larger muscle group	• Least intense • Single joint • Static • Small muscle • Simple

Learn More: Advanced Concepts of Personal Training Textbook p. 315

EXERCISE ORDER

1. Power Clean	85% 1RM	Fast, Heavy, Complex	P,P,P
2. Back Squat	85% 1RM	Heavy, Unstable, Cross joint	P,P,S
3. Walking Barbell Lunges	70% 1RM	Unstable, Difficult, Cross joint	P,P,S
4. Romanian Deadlift	75% 1RM	Cross joint, Large muscle	S,S
5. Overhead Lateral Squat	30% 1RM	Unstable, Dynamic but light	S,S
6. Unilateral Leg Curls	75% 1RM	Single Joint, Static	A,A

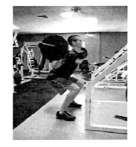 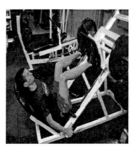 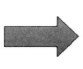 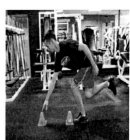

PRACTICE EXERCISE 8: EXERCISE ORDER
Place a number next to the exercise so it is put in proper order for a workout bout.

Hypertrophy

2	Bench press	3x10 75% 1RM (150 lbs.)
4	Lat pulldown	3x12 70% 1RM (90 lbs.)
3	Military press	3x10 70% 1RM (80 lbs.)
1	Squat	3x12 70% 1RM (175 lbs.)
5	Cable trunk rotation	3x12 50% 1RM (25 lbs.)

Back/Leg Strength

2	Weighted pull-ups	3x8 80% 1RM (BW + 20lbs.)
3	Unilateral leg press	3x8 per leg 75% (150 lbs.)
4	Machine leg curl	3x10 70% (60 lbs.)
5	Single arm row	3x10 72% (55 lbs.)
1	Deadlift	3x7 82.5% (205 lbs)

PROGRESSIONS

- Increase difficulty by changing a parameter of the movement
- Use the training variables to apply formatted overload
- Select training variables based on goal oriented outcomes

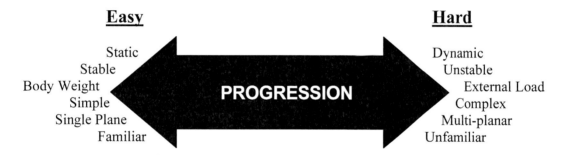

Learn More: Advanced Concepts of Personal Training Textbook p. 319

PROGRESSIVE OVERLOAD CONSIDERATIONS

- If **speed** of movement **increases** the **resistance** used **decreases**
- If the **stability** of movement **decreases** the **resistance decreases**
- If the **stability** is **decreased** and **velocity increased**, **resistance** must be further **decreased**

MOVEMENT PROGRESSIONS

- Establish starting points based on evaluative criteria
- Skill acquisition – begin with no resistance and change environments to maximize neuromuscular efficiency until skill is mastered
- Add resistance – base load assignments on phase of training and goals
- Add a level of difficulty by changing the movement environment – decrease load to accommodate compounding difficulty
- Increase difficulty based on desired response (speed, stability, resistance, complexity)

Easy/Simple

Bodyweight Movement
Forward Lunge
(Skill Acquisition)

Resisted Movement
Forward Lunge w/resistance
(Resisted Movement)

Bodyweight + Mild Instability
Walking Forward Lunge
(Dynamic)

Added Resistance + Mild Instability
MB Overhead Forward Lunge
(More Dynamic, Added Difficulty)

Movement Complexity
Forward Lunge w/MB rotation
(Dynamic Weighted, and Complex)

Hard/Complex

PROGRAMMING EXERCISE

CREATING THE PRESCIPTION

- Identify the key program needs
- Evaluate the findings and prioritize the need
- Identify general remedies to address the needs
- Select activities that match the participant's capabilities
- Combine activities to maximize attainable work
- Implement systems of training and exercise principles
- Determine the training cycle length
- Premeditate progressive overload

Learn More: Advanced Concepts of Personal Training Textbook p. 485

STEP 1. DATA COLLECTION

Identify key program needs using:

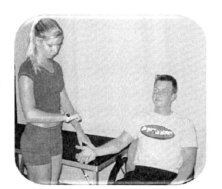

1 • Screening forms – HSQ and Behavior Questionnaire
2 • Resting test battery
3 • Physical fitness tests
4 • Participant interview (personal goals)

STEP 2. DEFINING NEED

Evaluate the findings and prioritize need:

1. Current disease or limiting health problem
2. Risk for limitations, disease, or health problem
3. Areas of lowest fitness level of health
4. Activity limiting factors
5. Areas that affect multiple outcomes
6. Performance, fitness, and vanity goals

STEP 3. NEEDS ANALYSIS

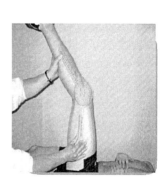

Hypertension	Blood pressure 160/92 mmHg
Pre-Diabetes	Blood glucose 110 mg/dl
Body Fat	20%
Low Back Pain	Intermittent lateral lumbar region
Muscle Imbalances	Shoulder, trunk, hip and knee
Poor Flexibility	Hamstring, gluteals, internal shoulder rotation, trunk extension and rotation
Cardiovascular Efficiency	33 ml/kg/min
Muscular Fitness	Deconditioned

STEP 4. PROGRAM CONSIDERATION PROCESS

Identify the Problem and match with Remedy or solution

PROBLEM	REMEDY
Hypertension	weight loss, aerobic training, diet *(handwritten)*
Pre-diabetes	Weight loss, increase total body activity
High body fat	*max caloric expenditure* diet, aerobic training, resistance training, *circuit training (handwritten)*
Low back pain	*dynamic Flexibility, improve ROM, trunk/hip muscle balance (handwritten)*
Muscle imbalance	Specific strengthening activities
Low CV fitness	*aerobic training DAILY (handwritten)*
Postural weakness	Total body strengthening activities
Poor flexibility	Increase ROM in deficient areas

STEP 5. SELECT ACTIVITIES

- Weight Loss – high caloric expenditure, highest attainable volume of work (circuits and supersets)
- Improve CRF – aerobic training (intervals and circuits)
- Improve Flexibility – dynamic and static stretching
- Increased Strength – pyramids, compound total body resistance training

STEP 6. SELECT "fixer" EXERCISES

Tight hip flexors	Single leg squat – *bulgarian squats (handwritten)*
Weak/tight abdominals	Step back to overhead reach
Tight glutes	*single leg crossover → Reverse lunge (handwritten)*
Tight hamstrings	*MB Goodmorning → Split stance RDL (handwritten)*
Tight trunk rotators	*lunge with rotation → any diagonal movement without moving hips. (handwritten)*

- Trainers should ensure that every activity serves a goal-specific function and addresses a need

MULTIPLE OUTCOMES

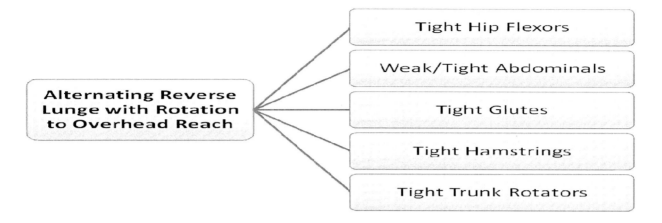

Alternating Reverse Lunge with Rotation to Overhead Reach
- Tight Hip Flexors
- Weak/Tight Abdominals
- Tight Glutes
- Tight Hamstrings
- Tight Trunk Rotators

STEP 7. MAKE INDIVIDUAL CONSIDERATIONS

- Specific Need: Does this exercise promote the desired outcome response? What is the purpose?
- Individual Capabilities: Can it be done safely and effectively?
- Movement Experience: How long will it take to teach?
- Fitness Level: How hard can they be challenged?
- Movement Aptitude: Is this exercise appropriate for this individual and the current training cycle?
- Limiting Factors: Is flexibility or back pain an issue?
- Goals: Is the exercise reflective of training goals and does it complement other training factors?
- Interests: Will they enjoy it?

PRESCRIPTION MATRIX

- Categorizes the training session by need, energy sequence, and order of operations
- Identify components of the exercise prescription
- Select the correct exercises and training systems to match the desired effects and needs

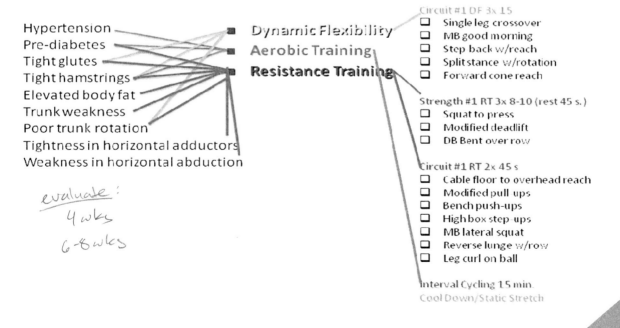

Hypertension
Pre-diabetes
Tight glutes
Tight hamstrings
Elevated body fat
Trunk weakness
Poor trunk rotation
Tightness in horizontal adductors
Weakness in horizontal abduction

Dynamic Flexibility
Aerobic Training
Resistance Training

Circuit #1 DF 3x 15
- ❑ Single leg crossover
- ❑ MB good morning
- ❑ Step back w/reach
- ❑ Split stance w/rotation
- ❑ Forward cone reach

Strength #1 RT 3x 8-10 (rest 45 s.)
- ❑ Squat to press
- ❑ Modified deadlift
- ❑ DB Bent over row

Circuit #1 RT 2x 45 s
- ❑ Cable floor to overhead reach
- ❑ Modified pull-ups
- ❑ Bench push-ups
- ❑ High box step-ups
- ❑ MB lateral squat
- ❑ Reverse lunge w/row
- ❑ Leg curl on ball

Interval Cycling 15 min.
Cool Down/Static Stretch

evaluate:
4 wks
6-8 wks

RESISTANCE TRAINING PRACTICAL

LOWER BODY TRAINING

Techniques

(1) Back squat	Front squat	Overhead squat	Single leg squat
(2) Deadlift	Modified deadlift	RDL	
(3) Static lunge	Forward lunge	Reverse lunge	Lateral lunge
(4) Step-up	Lateral step-up		

Learn More: Personal Training Technique & Assessment DVD Video

UPPER BODY TRAINING

Techniques

(1) Chest press	Chest fly	Close grip bench	Push-ups
(2) Military press	DB overhead press	Arnold press	
(3) Front raise	Side raise	Posterior raise	
(4) Bent-over row	Single arm row	Lat pull-down (explain)	Seated row (explain)
(5) Supine triceps ext.	Bicep curl	Hammer curls	

Learn More: Personal Training Technique & Assessment DVD Video

SAMPLE FUNCTIONAL TRAINING EXERCISES

Techniques

OH forward/reverse lunge	Forward lunge with press	Reverse lunge with rotation
Walking lunges with rotation	Single leg squat with frontal raise	Lateral squat swings
Overhead lateral lunge	Single leg marching T-raises	Dumbbell side reaches